PDQ
EVIDENCE-BASED
PRINCIPLES AND
PRACTICE

Second Edition

ANN McKIBBON, MLS, PhD
NANCY WILCZYNSKI, MSc, PhD
Health Information Research Unit
Department of Clinical Epidemiology and Biostatistics
McMaster University
Hamilton, Ontario, Canada

with

Angela Eady, BA, MLS and Susan Marks, BA, BEd

2009
PEOPLE'S MEDICAL PUBLISHING HOUSE
SHELTON, CONNECTICUT

People's Medical Publishing House
2 Enterprise Drive, Suite 509
Shelton, CT 06484
Tel: 203-402-0646
Fax: 203-402-0854
E-mail: info@pmph-usa.com

09 10 11 12/PMPH/9 8 7 6 5 4 3 2 1

ISBN 978-1-60795-006-6
Printed in China by People's Medical Publishing House
Copyeditor/Typesetter: Newgen; Cover designer: Mary McKeon

Sales and Distribution

Canada
McGraw-Hill Ryerson Education
Customer Care
300 Water St
Whitby, Ontario L1N 9B6
Canada
Tel: 1-800-565-5758
Fax: 1-800-463-5885
www.mcgrawhill.ca

Foreign Rights
John Scott & Company
International Publisher's Agency
P.O. Box 878
Kimberton, PA 19442
USA
Tel: 610-827-1640
Fax: 610-827-1671

Japan
United Publishers Services Limited
1-32-5 Higashi-Shinagawa
Shinagawa-ku, Tokyo 140-0002
Japan
Tel: 03-5479-7251
Fax: 03-5479-7307
Email: kakimoto@ups.co.jp

United Kingdom, Europe, Middle East, Africa
McGraw Hill Education
Shoppenhangers Road
Maidenhead
Berkshire, SL6 2QL
England
Tel: 44-0-1628-502500
Fax: 44-0-1628-635895
www.mcgraw-hill.co.uk

Singapore, Thailand, Philippines, Indonesia,
Vietnam, Pacific Rim, Korea
McGraw-Hill Education
60 Tuas Basin Link
Singapore 638775

Tel: 65-6863-1580
Fax: 65-6862-3354
www.mcgraw-hill.com.sg

Australia, New Zealand
Elsevier Australia
Tower 1, 475 Victoria Avenue
Chatswood NSW 2067
Australia
Tel: 0-9422-8553
Fax: 0-9422-8562
www.elsevier.com.au

Brazil
Tecmedd Importadora e Distribuidora
de Livros Ltda.
Avenida Maurilio Biagi 2850
City Ribeirao, Rebeirao, Preto SP
Brazil
CEP: 14021-000
Tel: 0800-992236
Fax: 16-3993-9000
Email: tecmedd@tecmedd.com.br

India, Bangladesh, Pakistan, Sri Lanka, Malaysia
CBS Publishers
4819/X1 Prahlad Street 24
Ansari Road, Darya, New Delhi-110002
India
Tel: 91-11-23266861/67
Fax: 91-11-23266818
Email:cbspubs@vsnl.com

People's Republic of China
PMPH
Bldg 3, 3rd District
Fangqunyuan, Fangzhuang
Beijing 100078
P.R. China
Tel: 8610-67653342
Fax: 8610-67691034
www.pmph.com

Contents

299709946

Foreword

Much has happened since the first edition of this manual a decade ago, and much of it is potentially good for helping people with health care problems. Biomedical and health care research are producing a geyser of new knowledge about the cause, course, diagnosis, prevention and treatment of health care problems, with many life-saving and life-enhancing remedies. The predicament that has emerged and continues to perplex is this: most care givers and patients can't readily access, accurately interpret, and appropriately apply this font of knowledge. This predicament is not just due to the volume and complexity of good health research, but also to the fact that important new knowledge is diluted beyond recognition by half-baked, misleading, dangerous, and very noisy information from explorations, "experts," and entrepreneurs. Add to this the troubles that practitioners have in learning new ways of doing things when they are beyond their formal training, and that all people have in learning new habits or eradicating bad habits, and you have a recipe for tragedy: only a tiny fraction of medical discovery is ever harnessed, and much of what is accomplished is offset by harms from tests and treatments that should have been abandoned long ago.

The principles and practice of evidence-based health care attempt to enable effective and consistent translation of knowledge from research into improved health care. The basic steps include appraising evidence reports, typically in the form of journal articles; interpreting the best available evidence in the context of individual patient's circumstances, wishes, and actions; informing policy makers and managers about the decisions they will need to make about the organization and quality of health services; and being able to quickly find current best evidence when it is needed.

This book chronicles the advances in evidence-based principles and practice. It provides a plain-language and balanced approach to understanding the basic principles of evidence generation and application, with special and detailed expertise in how to find studies that should be considered in addressing clinical questions.

v

The authors are trail blazers in the management of health research evidence. They have designed, conducted, reported, appraised, and disseminated research evidence for many years. Furthermore, they have pioneered and guided the development of techniques to track down the current best evidence concerning health care problems. Everyone can use these techniques if they master the concepts in this book. These concepts are described in an engaging and straightforward fashion, and readers will be well served by embracing the lessons with a view to becoming adept.

R. Brian Haynes, MD, PhD, FRSC
Professor of Clinical Epidemiology and Medicine
Chief, Health Information Research Unit
McMaster University
Hamilton, Ontario, Canada

Preface

Our exposure to evidence-based health care (EBHC) principles started in the late 1970s before the term was coined. We worked closely with many of the clinicians involved in the development of EBHC. Our involvement concentrated on the "information science" aspects of applying strong evidence to clinical decision making. Our work helped produce some of the first evidence-based journals: *ACP Journal Club, Evidence-Based Medicine, Evidence-Based Nursing, and Evidence-Based Mental Health*. Additionally, we did informatics research under the auspices of Brian Haynes, the chief of the Health Information Research Unit. This research has produced many findings and products. The Clinical Queries in PubMED and Ovid databases and the EvidenceUpdates and its complementary services are some that we hold as being important milestones in our careers.

Along the way we have raised children and once our parenting was well established we completed PhDs. Ann was first in 2005. Her PhD is in medical informatics from the University of Pittsburgh. She studied how clinicians use information resources in relation to their attitudes toward risk and uncertainty. Nancy followed suit in 2007 with a PhD in research methods from McMaster University. Her dissertation work centered on search filters for methods and content. The findings from her research (38 peer-reviewed articles) were the impetus for us to produce a new edition of our first PDQ book. We have learned much since 1999. The new edition is quite different from the first. We hope that what we see as improvements prove to be valuable for you.

We have kept the 2 main objectives of the first edition. First, we want to increase your knowledge and comfort with EBHC theory and principles. The people we have targeted in both editions are librarians and other information science people who deal with the information aspects of health care. We also feel that health professionals who seek a "gentle" introduction to EBHC principles can also learn much about research methods from reading and studying this book. The content will provide both the information professional and the clinician with a richer understanding of how health care research/evidence affects their daily work. It will also be a strong foundation for you when it comes time to make important health care decisions for yourself and the family and friends who are close to you.

Our second goal is to enhance your clinical information retrieval skills. With an understanding of how health care research is done and reported, you have a much easier task and become more effective at obtaining relevant material from the 4 major health databases: MEDLNE, EMBASE, CINAHL, and PsycINFO. The health care literature is vast. It includes material that is important to many audiences. Only a small proportion of the health care literature—often in the range of 1 item or article per 1000 published—is ready for direct clinical application. To put it another way, only a small portion of the published literature should change clinical practice. The laboratory and animal studies are important for health care researchers but they hold very little information that is useful for making decisions in clinical situations. We have reduced the amount of information we included on the indexing of specific articles in the databases because we now have empirically derived and validated search filters for most categories of articles.

With the reduction of searching examples, we have also increased our coverage of the research methods content. We have observed that information professionals and health care personnel have grown in their knowledge and skill in relation to EBHC. Schools are teaching more EBHC and continuing formal and informal education has played a role in advancing research methods knowledge for many of us already in practice. All of the chapters have been rewritten with special emphasis on new examples. Even more important, we have expanded the content to reflect the increased knowledge of our readers and the advances in EBHC that have happened in the past 10 years. We have also added 4 chapters while enhancing the existing 9 chapters. The new chapters are

- Clinical Prediction Guides

- Decision Analyses

- Differential Diagnosis and Disease Manifestation

- Secondary Publications: Health Technology Assessment

Other features that we have kept from the first edition include information on the history of clinical research and publishing. We have shortened this material, however, to include more of the important advances in EBHC theory and application. We have retained and updated the searching exercises at the end of chapters and have tried to show the range of material in all of the 4 databases. For the non-librarian audience, MEDLINE is the largest and most mature health database with almost 17 million citations. It is the only database of health care literature we include that is available at no cost through the PubMed interface. MEDLINE is funded by the U.S.

National Library of Medicine and therefore has content that is weighted toward being U.S. and medically based. EMBASE is a commercial database with emphasis on medical literature and allied health literature with a strong European flavor. It is produced in the Netherlands. It is marginally smaller than MEDLINE but is still a huge database. CINAHL (Cumulated Index to the Nursing and Allied Health Literature) concentrates on the non-medical health care literature. It is also astonishing rich in links to full text of the articles, documents, and scales. It also often includes the bibliography of articles in addition to the abstracts. PsycINFO is the online version of *Psychological Abstracts*. As its name implies, it covers all aspects of mental health and psychology/psychiatry. CINAHL and PsycINFO also include books and book chapters and theses and dissertations. MEDLINE and EMBASE do not include these items. People who wish to have access to the latter 3 resources must have institutional access to the databases or pay substantial personal subscriptions.

We have also kept and often enhanced our sections on the statistics and numbers associated with the various categories of research. Many people "dislike" statistics but some understanding of how numbers are used in health research studies and articles makes appreciation of the knowledge easier and more meaningful. We encourage you to do some "struggling" with the numerical concepts we have presented. Any understanding you have will only improve your ability and comfort in EBHC principles.

ACKNOWLEDGMENTS

We would not be writing this book without the myriad of people we have encountered during our journey at McMaster University. We tried to name those people important to us in our first edition. This time around we are not going to try to list important people except to say a special thank you to Brian Haynes who has inspired and challenged us to learn and grow—and get our PhDs. We also must acknowledge our work peers—Susan Marks and Angela Eady who again have rewritten their chapters on qualitative studies and economic analyses. Cindy Walker Dilks has been a wonderful peer on our career journeys. We miss you, Cindy.

Ann is nearing the time to think seriously about retirement. During the rewriting of this book she has constantly been reminded of the young librarians and information professionals who are being educated in new ways and starting out on exciting new careers. Her daughter Meghan Gamsby is one of these librarians. Meghan has read and commented on all of our chapters. The book is stronger because of her insights. I (Ann) dedicate this book, or at least my portion of it, to Meghan and her peers. You will take us far in the next generation of information professionals. I am very proud of you.

Nancy is continuing her research in the Health Information Research Unit at McMaster University. Exciting times lie ahead for all of us in the field of knowledge translation. Working on this book with Ann McKibbon, Susan Marks, and Angela Eady was a pleasure. I (Nancy) would like to thank Ann for including me as an author on the second edition of her book. I continue to learn a great deal from Ann. She is an excellent teacher. I dedicate my portion of this book to my family, Jerry, Jeffrey and Stephen. You have always provided ongoing support and unwavering encouragement.

AM
NW
January 2009

1

Introduction

Ann McKibbon

Health care professionals and librarians have recognized the reality of the information explosion for many years. Advances in technology, software, and the Internet give the impression that the explosion is gaining in force and magnitude. A major motivation for the development of online databases such as MEDLINE was to have better control of literature and information. This motivation remains only partly realized; we do not necessarily have better control—we just have faster access to more information. These are exciting and challenging times for all those interested in information access. New tools and skills are being developed, and more are needed to meet our information processing challenges. As a consequence, health care professionals and those in the information business cannot rely on the information and skills they learned during their schooling and must refresh their research skills and understanding of technology.

Evidence-based medicine (EBM), an approach to selecting and integrating the best available evidence into health care, has been advocated since the early 1980s as probably the most effective way to keep clinicians up to date and thus improve health care.[1-3] A large component of EBM practice includes harnessing the health care literature as the basis for practice decisions. The evidence in the literature is integrated with the patient's unique situation and values and the clinician's experience and education to come to the best possible care decision. Although medicine was one of the first disciplines to adopt these principles, other health disciplines have also espoused the principles and processes. Evidence-based nursing, mental health, dentistry, and alternative medicine have been recognized in the literature. We will use the general terms of evidence-based practice (EBP) or evidence-based health care (EBHC) to cover discussions of all disciplines unless we are discussing a specific discipline. In addition, we will use the terms "clinician" and "health care professional" to encompass all those who help patients and families make appropriate health care and related decisions: physicians, nurses, dentists, clergy, physical and occupational therapists, psychologists, midwives, and so on.

EVIDENCE-BASED HEALTH CARE DEFINITION

Evidence-based health care is a process of health care decision making and related behavior. Several definitions have developed. Definition one[1] states that clinicians who practice EBHC build on existing clinical experience and formal education (knowledge of pathophysiology and mechanisms of action) to integrate current evidence from the published literature into the patient care situation. Experience and basic knowledge are necessary, but not sufficient, for the practice of EBHC. Clinicians need to ground their practice in knowledge and fundamental principles and then base their decisions and actions on appropriate evidence from health care research, taking into account the unique needs and situation of the patient. Evidence can be from either original studies or trials or evidence-based secondary sources, such as systematic review articles and meta-analyses, decision analysis tools, clinical practice guidelines, and economic analyses. Definition one also emphasizes that knowing how to use the literature is imperative for ensuring that clinicians are providing optimal care.

According to definition two, EBHC "is the process of systematically finding, appraising, and using contemporaneous research findings as the basis for clinical decisions."[2] The key idea here is use of research findings (evidence) that are currently the best available. EBHC means a strong commitment to keeping up-to-date with changing and improving health care innovations reported in the literature. Lacking, or at least not explicit in this definition, is that the patient involved in the decision must be recognized as having his or her own needs, expectations, culture, spiritual beliefs, and preferences as well as situation. The patient him- or herself should be a partner in the decision-making process and completing care. Clinical setting, resources, practical implications, and cost constraints must also be considered.

Definition three is the one most often used in describing EBHC.[3] It reads:

... the conscientious, explicit, and judicious use of current best evidence in making decisions about the care of individual patients.

This definition implies conscious choice on the part of the clinician and patient, explicit and exact decisions being made and carried out, and always wisdom, experience, and judgment used to evaluate and apply this evidence. An individual patient with a specific need or problem is almost always involved in EBHC although decisions based on groups of people can be considered.

Evidence-based public health care applies to decision making for populations versus individuals; for example, the decision to immunize all students in a given school if a classmate is diagnosed with meningitis or how best to determine the presence of an outbreak important to the community.

While working with the material in this book, think carefully about your own discipline and job situation. For example, librarians can consider EBP in relation to their work with clinicians as well as for their own professional experience—evidence-based library and information practice.

FIVE STEPS OF EVIDENCE-BASED HEALTH CARE

EBHC is a 5-step process and each step takes time and energy. All 5 steps can take up to an hour or longer to complete, depending on the complexities and access to the original studies. The first step is **defining the question** that needs to be answered: this is often more difficult than first envisioned. Librarians often equate this step with the "reference interview" process that takes place each time a person asks for library assistance.

The second step is **collecting evidence to answer the question**. This is the step in which librarians can (and should) play a key role. This role can involve the provision of the evidence itself, or teaching clinicians and clinicians-in-training how to effectively and efficiently find evidence in the health care literature. More information resources are being produced that concentrate on providing ready-for-clinical-application evidence—things like evidence-based textbooks and web sites that summarize the findings of trials and studies along with actions for clinicians to take.

The third and fourth steps are the ones that utilize basic knowledge and previous clinical experience. The third step is the formal evaluation of the evidence that is gathered. This step is also called **critical appraisal**—the reading and extraction and analysis of the findings of the studies identified, taking into account the patient, setting, situation, and problem as defined in step one (the question). Fourth is the **integration of the evidence and patient factors** to make and carry out the decision. In many instances this fourth step is one of the most difficult to achieve. Some researchers label this step as "knowledge translation"—how to get the evidence applied or used.

The fifth step, one often omitted, is the **evaluation of the whole process** with a view to improving it the next time the EBHC cycle is followed. This 5-step process is almost identical to the information literacy process.[4] An overarching goal of many universities and colleges is to graduate students who are information literate.

Clinicians who espouse EBHC principles do not use the 5 steps for every health care encounter. Often the full 5-step process is done once or twice a week to address a specific question that the clinician feels needs consideration. An example of this would be a general internist who has noticed several new studies of drugs for congestive heart failure. At home one evening she mentally reviews the 3 patients she has seen that day, and is worried about 1 patient who does not seem to be responding to the usual drug regimen. She wonders if she should change or update her prescribing for this patient's congestive heart failure, which is complicated by insulin-dependent diabetes mellitus and poor adherence to medication regimes and lifestyle challenges. She determines the question she wishes to address, does a literature search, reads 2 high-quality articles assessing the new drugs, and decides that this patient's amiodarone dose probably should be changed.

Because of this review of new drugs for congestive heart failure, the clinician has confirmed that her care for these patients is not quite current and appropriate. She then changes her general approach to prescribing for those patients who have congestive heart failure. As this pattern of several EBHC cycles per week is followed, most of the common situations a clinician encounters will be addressed and updated if needed. Clinicians can, however, never be completely current, especially when patients present with diseases or conditions that are uncommon in their normal practice. EBHC "allows" that clinicians cannot know or be current on everything while providing mechanisms for helping them give the best care they can for the majority of their patients. Good clinicians know their own abilities and when to treat or refer patients.

CRITICISMS

As with any new development, EBHC has its detractors. Criticisms need to be evaluated to ascertain if refinements or improvements are needed. Much wisdom and understanding is often gained by a thorough and honest evaluation of others' reactions, comments, and criticisms. The Lancet's editors[5] accused EBHC proponents of being subversive, narrow, and lacking finesse, with the "evidence-based movement" having certain similarities to fundamentalist cults. Any new movement includes individuals who are excited and want to quickly and completely change existing behavior and practice. In addition, movements often start with a simplistic "black-and-white" view of reality, which matures and becomes more complex as truly beneficial features of the movement become incorporated into routine use. If these 2 features of EBHC are true, then The Lancet editors are probably right in their assessment. EBHC will, however, grow and mature as it becomes incorporated into the fabric of health care.

In a more gentle but substantive critique, Feinstein and Horowitz[6] point out that the "laudable goal of making clinical decisions based on evidence" must be tempered by 3 additional truths. The first, and probably most important, is that each patient brings his or her own situation, preferences, culture, and needs to the situation, all of which must be balanced with the evidence. Second, today's golden truth may easily be tomorrow's inaccurate, or even inappropriate, information. The third, many of our current best-care practices have not and never will be evaluated using the best of EBHC approaches.

Several reasons account for this absence of evaluation in some situations. For example, ethics do not allow researchers to withhold blood transfusions from accident victims to test if the transfusions will save lives. They also cannot decline fluids from young infants who are dehydrated merely for testing purposes. Common sense tells us that children should wear mittens when they go out in the snow and sky divers should use parachutes, even though these situations have not been formally studied in large-scale trials. Funding agencies are not interested in financing large-scale studies on topics such as the removal of ear wax. Other examples of these "gray areas" of practices that are not solidly evaluated are the use of some well-established antibiotics for infections, antidepressants for depression, implantable pacemakers for symptomatic heart block, and catheterization for urinary obstruction.

COMMUNICATION AND RESEARCH

The rest of this chapter gives a brief historic background of biomedical communication and research. The book then provides a broad overview of how current biomedical research is conducted, reported, and used by health professionals. It includes 8 major primary clinical research types: therapy, diagnosis, etiology and causation, prognosis and natural history, economics, clinical prediction rules, differential diagnosis and disease manifestations, and qualitative research (understanding the processes of disease and health). The basic methodologies unique to each research type, along with examples of strong research, are provided. The secondary EBHC literature (systematic review articles, clinical practice guidelines, health technology assessments, and decision analyses) are also studied. Each chapter also includes information on how indexers index articles of each type of research, and how this indexing can be used along with abstracts and title words to retrieve ready-for-clinical-application material for each type from the large biomedical databases.

A combination of approaches for each research area is used to develop methodological filters for MEDLINE, CINAHL, PsycINFO, and EMBASE searching using clinical examples. When to use this methodological filtering is discussed, and sample questions are included at the end of each chapter. The appendix includes several proposed answers from various databases for each clinical question.

HISTORY OF SCIENTIFIC COMMUNICATION

EBHC has its roots in ancient history. Men and women have always strived to learn, experiment, and pass on their knowledge and experience. To properly understand modern health care research, one needs to start with a review of the historical process of scientific communication and its various stages of development.

Oral Tradition

Story telling and the oral tradition were the first methods used to communicate, teach, and pass on knowledge and skills. Story telling was the main form of scientific communication for many centuries. The oral tradition for transfer of health care information is still used in many cultures today, either formally through village healers in less developed countries, or through the handing-down of home or folk remedies from one generation to another, often through the women in a family. Oral communication of health care information is also used during morning hospital reports, case presentations, and patient history taking. Formal communication of scientific ideas now encompasses much more than the oral traditions.

Letters

Writing developed 5000 years ago,[7] and several centuries later the Greeks and Romans were writing letters. Soon letters were routinely exchanged by philosophers, mathematicians, and other thinkers. Archimedes and Ptolemy were among the first to write to their acquaintances, telling them of their scientific ideas and theories. Letters began the tradition of formal, recorded modes of scientific communication, and this continued for many centuries.

Handwritten Books

Handwritten letters soon evolved into handwritten books. These were valuable to the few people who could read them. The library in ancient Alexandria was legendary for its collection of medical texts, and when it was destroyed much knowledge was lost. Copies of medical texts were kept by the monasteries, and they were often tended with as much care as religious texts.

Printing Press and Books

The next major advance in scientific communication was the development of the printing press more than 500 years ago in Germany. The first illustrated medical textbook was printed in 1495 in Venice. Johannes de Ketham, author of *Fasciculus Medicine,* included descriptions of various common diagnostic and therapeutic procedures such as blood letting, urine examination, pregnancy care, and behavior during epidemics. Medical books continued to be important to clinicians and libraries for many centuries for communicating both new and established health knowledge.

Guild System and Journals

In the 1600s the guild system became part of the fabric of industry, technology, and science. Scientists established their own societies and soon started writing short communications for presentation at society meetings. These short pieces were subsequently printed in publications such as *Philosophical Transactions* and *Transactions of the Royal Society of London*. These collections of short presentations became the first journals. As journals spread, books provided less *new* information and became tools that *integrate* knowledge, resulting in the textbooks, handbooks, and encyclopedias we have today.

Printed Indexes

Several hundred years later, researchers and health care professionals still rely on journal articles for communication of ideas and advancements. Indexing and abstracting services such as *Index Medicus* and *Chemical Abstracts* were developed around the turn of the 19th century, when the number of journals grew so large that formal indexing systems were required to determine what had been published and where. *Index Medicus*, developed by John Shaw Billings, a U.S. surgeon, was one of the first indexes of the medical literature. *Cumulative Index to Nursing and Allied Health Literature* was started by the early 1940s to index the nursing literature. The original 3-by-5-inch card file that was the basis of the nursing index still exists.

Computer Databases

Computerized versions of these indexes were developed starting in the late 1960s. Computer tapes of the bibliographic information were first made to speed the publication of printed indexes, but developers soon realized that the computer tapes used in typesetting could be harnessed to provide searching capabilities. Early computerized retrieval searching systems were batch-mode processes that required long turnaround times. Teletype machines with paper tape output and acoustic couplers were the next advances in the early days of online searching. The staff at the U.S. National Library of Medicine required that searchers pass a 4-month training course in MEDLINE search techniques before they were certified and allowed to search. This was soon reduced to a 2-4 week course. Shorter but mandatory training was still enforced well into the 1980s. Initially only librarians did online searching, but with the proliferation of computers and telecommunication networks, anyone with Internet access can and does use these systems. The public are now the heaviest users of MEDLINE.

The Internet

A huge volume of health care information is available on the Internet through full-text articles, blogs, web pages, etc. The quality of the information is difficult to evaluate and the peer review process that evaluates journal articles is not enforced. The Internet is, however, here to stay, but wisdom and skill are needed to use it effectively and evaluate the quality and usefulness of the information as well as keep up-to-date with advances. The current size and complexity of the literature means it is difficult to retrieve citations relevant to the question and appropriate for clinical decision making. Easy, fast, and efficient retrieval skills can be developed, however, if one understands how the health care literature is structured.

PUBLISHING WEDGE

The biomedical literature is hierarchical in nature, and includes many types or categories of journal articles. Figure 1-1 shows these categories and how they fit into a publishing and research hierarchy of 7 levels. Biomedical researchers and clinicians must use material from all 7 levels in their area of study, although researchers often specialize in material from one level or another. To illustrate this, imagine a basic researcher who works on an animal model for a specific disease, such as scrapie in sheep, a look-alike disease for multiple sclerosis. This researcher can concentrate on literature published in a narrow range of categories of information.

Clinicians, on the other hand, need to use information on treatments for many diseases or conditions, some of which have been firmly and convincingly proved, and some which are less certain as a basis for clinical decision making. The publishing wedge for therapy depicted in Figure 1-1 represents the structure of the health care literature that evaluates interventions. The wedge and its shape show both the types of publication and their relative numbers. All levels on the wedge are important to the process of discovering and proving health care treatment advances, but not all levels are equally useful for making patient care decisions. Other, similar wedges could be drawn for diagnostic and screening test evaluation, etiology and causation studies, prognosis and natural history questions, and economic analysis. From the top of the wedge, where numerous "ideas" papers exist, we move through a series of levels to the relatively few that report ready-for-application clinical research (the ones that are appropriate for EBHC decision making). The number of publications in each level decreases substantially, with, it is hoped, only the best from each level moving on to the next step.

Level 1: "Ideas" Papers

The first level in the publishing wedge includes "ideas" papers. Many are published in the health literature; they include such items as editorials, letters to the editor, and general "think" pieces, often with little hard evidence.

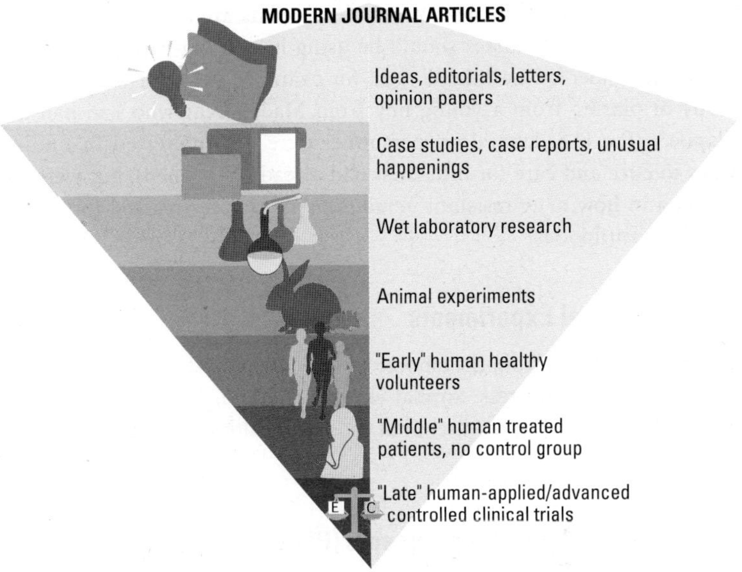

Figure 1-1. Publishing wedge for intervention trials.

Level 2: Case Reports

At the next broad level, ideas are discussed in relation to 1 or several patients: reports of single or a few cases (case studies) or of unusual happenings. The conclusions or assumptions made on the basis of these papers are often later rejected, but they are the papers we remember. One example that I remember is about "blue jeans thighs," which was identified when children with new, unwashed blue jeans, wet diapers, and discolored legs are brought to the emergency department by distraught parents.[9] A more serious example looks at the potential danger of scurvy caused by malnutrition in patients who have cancer. Fain et al describe 6 men who were diagnosed with scurvy from 1993 to 1996 among 3723 patients with cancer. All 6 improved dramatically after they were given vitamin C.[10] Because of this case report, clinicians who treat patients with cancer can be aware that this potentially serious disease can occur, and become vigilant for indications of scurvy.

Level 3: Laboratory Testing

Some of the ideas from the previous section or level will go on to wet laboratory testing: the test-tube-and-beaker stage. As with all levels, information and knowledge gained while evaluating the ideas in this level (the laboratory) are essential in health care research. If information from levels farther down the wedge is available, however, level 3 data are not the information that physicians and nurses should be using in making patient care decisions. The paper by Galimand et al, for example, describes a laboratory study of plasma from a young boy from Madagascar who had had the plague.[11] The U.S. laboratory personnel were not interested in finding ways to cure and care for him (that had already happened), but were interested in how drug-resistant *Yersinia pestis* isolates reacted to various standard antibiotics.

Level 4: Animal Experiments

Promising findings from the laboratory level are passed on to the next step in the evaluation process: animal experimentation. Not everyone agrees with using animals in research, but modern health care would be poorer without it.

Level 5: Early Human Experiments (Phase I Trials)

The 3 smaller (and lower) levels of the research wedge for therapies are devoted to evaluation in humans. Evaluations from the first level (also know as Phase I trials) study a limited number of humans, usually volunteers. These studies often include 5 to 15 individuals and last only a short time. Researchers often evaluate drugs or other interventions for obvious adverse effects. Marcurad et al studied healthy volunteers who were evaluated for their absorption of vitamin B12 after taking omeprazole.[12] The men studied had no clinical need to take the omeprazole, but researchers wanted to know about potential adverse effects. A general approximation is that Phase I trials take a year to plan, execute, and complete. Again, information proved from studies at this point in the research process is important to the whole research and evaluation cycle, but the clinical usefulness of the information is still limited.

Level 6: Case Series (Phase II Trials)

The second human therapy testing level is known as Phase II trials. In these studies, researchers often treat a small series of consecutive or carefully selected patients with an intervention such as surgery, counseling, or physical exercise programs. Often, no control or comparison group is included. An example of a study from this level of publication is one by Schumacher et al.[13] They evaluated 20 consecutive patients who were scheduled for triple coronary bypass surgery. When the grafting was done, a small amount of human growth factor was injected around the new vein to ascertain if the growth factor, an expensive drug, would help establish new capillaries and improve or speed return of cardiac function. At the end of the study more new capillaries than expected had grown around the graft in most patients. Phase II trials generally take 2 years from start to finish.

Sildenafil, or Viagra, was first developed as an antihypertensive agent; and it was at this Phase II stage of testing that researchers felt that the high blood pressure was not controlled effectively, and they chose to stop evaluating this drug for hypertension. The women in the study returned their unused medication as asked, but the men refused because of the side effects they had been experiencing. After questioning the men, researchers decided that sildenafil had other marketing possibilities, and its progression through the research wedge was recommenced, this time evaluating sildenafil for its ability to treat erectile dysfunction. The researchers moved back to the laboratory and animal levels before returning to human testing of sildenafil. As in the other levels in the wedge, the most promising articles move on to the next step in the research process.

Level 7: Clinical Trials (Phase III Trials)

The third level (Phase III trials) comprises the studies that EBHC practitioners advocate be used by health care professionals in making patient care decisions. These trials are often large and labor- and resource-intensive. They are the ones, however, that have enough "power" and design strength to separate true health care advances from those that produce more harm than good. The CLASP trial[14] was designed to answer the question of whether aspirin protects pregnant women with hypertension and their infants from the morbidity and mortality associated with pre-eclampsia and eclampsia. Both of these conditions are substantial problems in the developed world. Data from all 6 levels of the research wedge suggested that aspirin was a simple, effective, and low-cost treatment that could save lives and improve maternal and infant outcomes. These outcomes included seizures in the mother and low birth weight and intrauterine growth retardation in the infant. In the CLASP trial, 9362 pregnant women were studied; half received aspirin (60 mg per day) and half received placebo (an inert substance designed to seem like aspirin). When the data were analyzed, outcomes for women allocated to aspirin were shown to be equivalent to the outcomes for women who received placebo.

Calcium was also thought to be an important agent to improve maternal and infant health in pre-eclampsia and eclampsia. It, too, was shown to be ineffective in the large clinical trial (at this point of the wedge). Because of these 2 large studies, women at risk for high blood pressure in pregnancy are not routinely given aspirin or calcium to prevent pre-eclampsia and its related problems. Phase III trials often take a minimum of 3 years to complete, and require at least several hundreds of thousands of dollars to fund. Once completed, the results of the study can be assembled with other studies and the evidence submitted to agencies such as the U.S .Food and Drug

Administration. Once they are formally approved, the intervention can be implemented in clinical care.

Phase IV Trials

Phase IV trials are "beyond the point of the wedge," and are often called post-marketing studies. They are designed to evaluate the long-term safety and rare adverse effects, and sometimes the economics of drugs or interventions that have already been proved useful in Phase III trials. Long-term safety aspects are discussed in Chapter 2 (Therapy), adverse effects in Chapter 4 (Etiology), and economics has its own chapter (Chapter 12: Economics Analyses).

The discussion of the "intervention" wedge includes areas of therapy or treatment (e.g., is an antibiotic needed for recurrent otitis media?), quality improvement (e.g., will a computer-generated reminder increase the rate of signed advance directives by elderly patients?), and prevention and control (e.g., how can coronary vessels be kept free from restenosis after successful thrombolysis and angioplasty?). Besides the intervention wedge, wedges also exist for diagnostic or screening studies. For example, can we find a simple blood test to predict which patients in the emergency department with chest pain are having a myocardial infarction, so that those who need treatment receive it and those who are not having a myocardial infarction are evaluated correctly, reassured, and sent home or should we screen all adults for colorectal cancer using fecal occult blood tests. A wedge also exists for almost all other research domains.

The most important aspect of the material that is ready for clinical application is that the studies done here are comparative in nature. True proof of the benefit of a health care advance is if the comparative evidence shows improvements either in care or understanding of a disease or wellness situation.

Only approximately 1 idea in 5000 makes it through the testing for most areas of health care and becomes available for clinical application. In some areas of health care, such as cancer drugs, the differential is even greater. More than 40,000 potential drugs start at the top of the wedge for every drug that is evaluated and proven to be an effective cancer medication. Therefore, effective retrieval skills are vital for health care decision making. This book concentrates on understanding clinical trials and other study designs that form the body of evidence that EBHC practitioners advocate for use in making decisions (material at the point of the evidence wedge) and how they can be retrieved for application.

RESOURCES FOR CLINICAL STUDIES

It would be fairly simple for health care professionals to keep up to date if easy access to current best evidence for patient care existed in 1 source.

Journals that publish only reports of advanced tip-of-the-wedge research involving patients who are similar to their own *do not exist!* Haynes[15] has described and categorized the information needs and possibilities of information resources for clinicians. His categorization takes into account how the clinical information we describe in this book is presented in various products and services. Some information resources summarize studies of clinical interventions and provide how-to-apply information for clinicians. Some, like the MEDLINE database, provide nothing more than links to full-text articles or just citations to journal articles.

MEDLINE Filters

MEDLINE has limited use for clinicians because the database is so large and presents challenges in finding exactly what is needed for a given clinical situation. In conjunction with Brian Haynes of the McMaster University Health Information Research Unit, the authors have developed tools to make "clinical" retrieval from MEDLINE much faster and more effective.[16]

MEDLINE and other database searches are usually subject or content based. Content searching is done for drugs, diseases, syndromes, authors, and so on, with concepts put together in various Boolean operator (AND, OR, and NOT) combinations. These content-based searches do not differentiate among levels on the publication wedge—the idea paper, wet laboratory report, animal testing results, and human studies that include the content will all be retrieved. Subject searching is appropriate for research needs (e.g., retrieving everything on CD4+ cell counts predicting mortality in patients with AIDS), but *not* for clinical needs (e.g., several good papers on starting zidovudine combined with other drugs in patients with AIDS who have low CD4+ cell counts). The material at the point of the wedge (clinical trials) is unique in the methods that are used to conduct the research.

Searching in MEDLINE and other large databases can be harnessed to retrieve only citations of studies with a specific methodology. If we understand the basic methodologies of clinical research, we can go beyond simple subject or content searching. We can use strategies to retrieve only the articles that are ready-for-application (EBHC)—the ones at the narrowest point of the wedge, often referred to as clinical research. Each clinical category has its own research methods, and consequently its own retrieval strategies.

We undertook a study to determine if we could develop search filters or search hedges that could retrieve only those articles and ones like them— for example, all diagnosis or all therapy articles. With funding from the U.S. National Library of Medicine we did a hand search of 170 clinical journals. All of the ready-for-clinical-application studies were tagged for their category (therapy, diagnosis, etiology, prognosis, clinical prediction, economics, and systematic reviews and qualitative studies). Studies could have more than 1 category. Once these articles were tagged, we proceeded to develop and test the search filters. This project produced searching filters for therapy, diagnosis, etiology, prognosis, clinical prediction, qualitative, and economic studies as well as systematic reviews and clinical practice guidelines for MEDLINE, CINAHL, EMBASE, and PsycINFO where appropriate. Our search filters are available for use in PubMed through the Clinical Queries page (http://www.ncbi.nlm.nih.gov/entrez/query/static/clinical.shtml) and the Health Services Research Queries page (http://www.nlm.nih.gov/nichsr/hedges/search.html). They are also available for use in Ovid (http://gateway.ovid.com/) by limiting your search with any one of the Clinical Queries (after entering your disease content terms, click on Additional Limits and choose any one of the Clinical Queries). Additionally our search filters for MEDLINE and CINAHL are available through EBSCO (http://www.ebscohost.com/). These filters are an important foundation of the rest of the chapters in this book. A full listing of the methods and filters is available online.[16]

HISTORY OF CLINICAL RESEARCH

To understand clinical research it is useful to study its history and stages, as we did for scientific communication. Clinical research has a long history[17,18]; the first recorded clinical trial is in the Bible in Daniel 1:6 to 1:16. Grimes[19] assesses the strengths and weakness of this first trial of nutritional interventions using modern research standards. Daniel and his friends Shadrack, Meshach, and Abednego refused to eat food from the king's table as it was unclean, having been blessed by idols. They chose to eat other food and asked the overseers to compare their outcomes with other young men who did eat the king's food—a comparative trial of determining which foods are better. Grimes contends that this Babylonian trial was good research with flaws common even in studies today. Although his article is somewhat tongue-in-cheek, Grimes contends that the Daniel study has many strengths, including being comparative in nature with a contemporary (same time) control group (others in the court), blinded outcome assessment by the king, and the "striking brevity of the report." The weaknesses, according to Grimes, included a long lag time between execution of the study and its publication (100s of years), no randomization, and confounding of the study by divine intervention (see Chapter 2: Therapy for explanations of these terms).

Scurvy

The first reported controlled therapy trial took place in the United Kingdom in 1747. It was said to be controlled because Lind "controlled" who got what in his study to determine if any food or nutritional supplements could prevent or cure scurvy. Since the early 1600s, many people felt that citrus fruits might reduce the incidence of scurvy during long ocean voyages. Lind studied 12 sailors with scurvy, evaluating 6 potential treatments in comparison with one another. Two sailors were given sea water, 2 were given vinegar, 2 were given lemons and limes, 2 were given elixir vitriol (copper sulfate), 2 got a garlic and mustard mixture, and 2 were given cider. The sailors who received the citrus fruits recovered.[18] Although the results of this early trial were effective, low cost, and easy to implement, the innovation was not adopted by the British Navy until 1795. Once adopted the intervention helped Britain gain dominance over the seas.

Cold Vaccines

Methodologies have developed since the scurvy trial, and have matured quickly in the past several decades. The first modern U.S. comparative and controlled trial was published by Diehl et al in 1938.[20] They studied cold vaccines in 498 university students at the University of Minnesota. Half of the students received vaccinations and half received identical placebo injections. Both groups reported substantial reductions in the number of colds in the year after vaccination compared with the previous year. However, the incidence rates for colds were similar in both groups at the end of the trial. The vaccination research program continued over many years and throughout many trials, but cold vaccinations were never shown to be effective.

These controlled trials are strongest when the methods of putting people into study groups are without bias—in a strong comparison the groups should be as equal as possible at the start. This is usually achieved with randomization—the process of putting groups together solely by chance (e.g., flipping a coin). Historians cannot tell if the Minnesota trial was randomized, even after checking the original trial documents in the university archives and the historical collection of material at the U.S. National Library of Medicine. It was finally decided that this trial was not randomized. The first randomized controlled trial was done in Great Britain for tuberculosis.

Streptomycin for Tuberculosis

The first truly randomized controlled trial was done in the United Kingdom and published by the *British Medical Journal* in 1948. The British Medical Research Council's trial of streptomycin for tuberculosis[21] is considered a milestone in health care research. Interestingly, the impetus for the randomization in the 1948 streptomycin study did not come from the desire to advance scientific methodology, but because only half of the streptomycin needed for all patients with tuberculosis was available. The Medical Research Council staff felt that the fairest allocation method to decide who would receive the drug would be by chance alone, and therefore randomization to treatment groups was done (each person had a 50% chance of receiving streptomycin or the placebo). Streptomycin was shown to be effective in curing tuberculosis, and soon many sanatoriums were closed worldwide. This trial became the recognized standard for health care researchers and embodies many of the techniques, policies, and procedures used in current health care research.

Smoking and Lung Cancer

The *British Medical Journal* also published another research "first," this time in the area of etiology and causation. The question of cause-and-effect is an important one in health care, as are the questions of how to diagnose and treat diseases and conditions and understand their progression. One of the first well-done causation studies, published in 1950, formally assessed why the rates of lung cancer were increasing in England and Wales after World War II. Deaths from lung cancer had gone from 612 in 1922 to 9287 in 1947. Doll and Hill[22] studied general atmospheric pollution from the exhaust fumes of cars, the surface dust of tarred roads, and smoke and residue from industrial plants and coal fires, plus smoking. They developed a new study design, called a case-control study. "Cases," those with lung cancer, were matched and compared with "controls," those without lung cancer. The rates of exposure to the pollution and various kinds of smoke were compared in cases and controls, and conclusions drawn. By the end of their case-control study, Doll and Hill felt confident that tobacco smoking, and not tarred roads or industrial pollution, was associated with the large increase in lung cancer deaths. Both Doll and Hill were knighted for their innovative and groundbreaking work in the area of tobacco smoke pollution and also for their work improving and perfecting health care research methods. Both continued to produce high quality health care research and train many generations of British researchers.

Systematic Review Articles

One of the first studies to combine data from various trials—the forerunner of modern meta-analyses—is also from the *British Medical Journal*. Karl Pearson[23] published a report in 1904 that combined enteric fever statistics from several sources. He combined data from 4 reports of incidence data (new cases) from the British Army in South Africa and 1 from the British Army in India. For mortality, he added another set of data from South Africa. It is interesting that even though his article was short and included several tables and did not have an abstract, introduction, or references, it included a discussion of the ideas of homogeneity of the data (are the data similar enough to combine in 1 analysis?) and of weighting the values in the data sets by study size. Both concepts are vitally important to modern-day meta-analysts, and they are discussed in the first paragraph of Pearson's study. Karl Pearson was a well-known statistician and not a health care professional. He developed the Pearson coefficient that is widely used today, along with many other important statistical concepts and methodologies, although he is not recognized as a founder in the development of systematic review article methods.

U.S. Randomized Controlled Trial

One of the first large, multicenter, truly randomized controlled trials done in the United States was published in 1956. It studied the optimal usage and dose of oxygen in small and premature babies,[24] and is an example of working through the cycle of research from observation to proof of benefit or harm we have discussed. In the early 1950s, oxygen became easier to provide to hospitalized people and special care nurseries were using oxygen to save premature infants' lives. In practice, because of the effectiveness of the oxygen, nurses and physicians were using increasing concentrations of oxygen in their desire to save even more premature babies. The babies were alive, but in a 5-year period in the late 1940s and early 1950s, more than 10,000 U.S. babies had lost their sight. No one seemed to know why. Even the *Saturday Evening Post* tried to solve the mystery by commissioning and publishing a large investigative report. The observations were necessary but it took a well-done randomized controlled trial of different doses of oxygen by Kinsey et al many years after the blindness was first noted to solve the mystery. They completed and published a scientifically sound controlled and comparative dose-finding study to establish the best dose of oxygen that balanced the benefits and harms of the therapy. Oxygen is now used very carefully and only as needed—not routinely—in premature infants, and many fewer cases of blindness occur.

SUMMARY OF CURRENT CLINICAL RESEARCH

Health care research has continued to evolve in the past 50 to 60 years and each category of research has developed its own unique set of research methods and techniques. Two common features that apply to all clinical research studies are that they are comparative and preplanned. As previously stated, the first, and probably most important, aspect is that they are comparative. Without valid and reliable comparisons between 2 or more groups, health care would be driven by opinions, observations, and current procedures rather than by true scientific advances. An example of the comparisons for a therapy trial is a comparison of persons taking 1 drug with persons taking another drug or placebo (e.g., aspirin versus warfarin for stroke prevention in persons with atrial fibrillation). Treatment group (also called intervention or study group) participants are those who receive the active, new, or untested therapy. Control participants form the other comparison group(s).

Control patients usually get standard treatment (or no treatment) instead of the experimental therapy. In the oxygen trial described above, the groups of premature infants were formed and each obtained one of the levels of oxygen under study. At the end of the study the groups were analyzed and compared to determine rates of survival (the benefits of oxygen) and blindness (the harms of oxygen).

A diagnosis study will compare the results of 2 or more diagnostic tests in persons with and without the disease in question (e.g., thallium scanning versus cardiac enzyme measurements to assess whether patients who come to the emergency department with chest pain are actually having a myocardial infarction). An etiology and causation study compares persons exposed to some agent thought to cause a disease and those not exposed (e.g., very elderly persons, some with and some without high levels of cholesterol, who are then compared to ascertain if high cholesterol levels are associated with longer survival for persons over the age of 85; they seem to be). Another interesting causation question sorted out using comparative methods is the reason why librarians, like teachers and women physicians, have more breast cancer.[25] This increase in breast cancer seems to be related to postponing having children until later in life when their education is complete.

For prognosis and natural history studies, the comparative feature is present, but less evident. The comparison is best addressed by the example of a woman who has just been told that she has multiple sclerosis. She wants to know if this disease will affect her life style or survival compared with what could be expected if she did not have multiple sclerosis. Economic analyses compare costs of implementing a new procedure with costs if the procedure had not been implemented.

Careful, comprehensive planning goes into research studies before they start. Initially, a research question is posed that takes into account the patient's disease or condition, the procedure, duration, outcomes, and so on. From this question, protocols are developed that include very specific details describing all aspects of the study. For example, all drug studies include dosages, administration routes, and timing (e.g., 20 mg per day, 4 times daily, 1 hour before meals). They also include details for dealing with adverse reactions to the drugs, patient inclusion and exclusion criteria, how to encourage and measure patient adherence, how to deal with dropouts, what measures to use for evaluation, procedures for recruitment and follow up of all patients, and processes and timing for all final evaluations of all patients.

Diagnosis studies list in exact detail all procedures for the tests that are being studied (e.g., how to ask and score the 4 questions used in the CAGE questionnaire to identify problem drinking: have you ever tried to *Cut* down on your drinking, has anyone ever been *Angry* at your drinking, have you ever felt *Guilty* about your drinking, and have you ever needed an *Eye-opener*?). Causation studies define exposures (e.g., cigarette pack years) and outcomes. Prognosis studies define exact disease characteristics (e.g., first episode of optic neuritis of more than 1 week duration in 1 or both eyes) and the outcomes (e.g., multiple sclerosis based on magnetic resonance images of lesions on the brain within 5 to 10 years of optic neuritis).

In addition, all research studies use people who have or are at risk for the specific conditions, taking special care in ascertaining who should be studied and how they will be selected. Issues of funding, ethics, authorship, measurement of benefits and harms, and statistical and numerical data are also common across research studies.

Here the similarities among the types of research studies end. Each of the following chapters will discuss a specific type of research and what distinguishes it beyond the shared characteristics of being comparative and preplanned and the other issues just listed.

REFERENCES

1. Oxman AD, Sackett DL, Guyatt GH. Users' guides to the medical literature. I. How to get started. The Evidence-Based Medicine Working Group. *JAMA.* 1993;270:2093-2095.

2. Haynes RB, Sackett DL, Guyatt G,Tugwell P. *Clinical Epidemiology: How to do Clinical Practice Research.* 3rd ed. Lippincott, Williams and Wilkins. 2006.

3. Sackett DL, Rosenberg WM, Gray JA, et al. Evidence based medicine: what it is and what it isn't. *BMJ.* 1996;312:71-72.

4. Association of Colleges and Research Libraries. Information Literacy Competency Standards for Higher Education. American Library Association. 2007. Accessed August 11, 2008. http://www.ala.org/ala/acrl/acrlstandards/informationliteracycompetency.cfm

5. Evidence-based medicine in its place [editorial]. *Lancet.* 1995;346:785.

6. Feinstein AR, Horwitz RI. Problems in the "evidence" of "evidence-based medicine." *Am J Med.* 1997;103:529-535.

7. De Solla Price D. The development and structure of the biomedical literature. In: Warren K, ed. *Coping with the Biomedical Literature: A Primer for the Scientist and Clinician.* New York, NY: Praeger; 1981:3-16.

8. De Solla Price D. Communication in science: the ends—philosophy and forecast. In: De Reuck A, ed. *Communication in Science: Documentation and Automation.* London: Churchill; 1967:189-213.

9. Lantner RR, Ros SP. Blue jeans thighs. *Pediatrics.* 1991;88:417.

10. Fain O, Mathieu E, Thomas M. Scurvy in patients with cancer. *BMJ.*1998;316: 1661-1662.

11. Galimand M, Guiyoule A, Gerbaud G, et al. Multidrug resistance in *Yersinia pestis* mediated by a transferable plasmid. *N Engl J Med.* 1997;337:667-680.

12. Marcuard SP, Albernaz L, Khazanie PG. Omeprazole therapy causes malabsorption of cyanocobalamin (vitamin B12). *Ann Intern Med.* 1994;120: 211-215.

13. Schumacher B, Pecher P, von Specht BU, Stegmann T. Induction of neoangiogenesis in ischemic myocardium by human growth factors: first clinical results of a new treatment of coronary heart disease. *Circulation.* 1998;97:645-650.

14. CLASP: a randomised trial of low-dose aspirin for the prevention and treatment of preeclampsia among 9364 pregnant women. CLASP (Collaborative Low-dose Aspirin Study in Pregnancy) Collaborative Group. *Lancet.* 1994;343:619-629.

15. Haynes RB. Of studies, syntheses, synopses, summaries, and systems: the "5S" evolution of information services for evidence-based health care decisions. *ACP J Club.* 2006 Nov-Dec;145(3):A8.

16. Health Information Research Unit. McMaster University. HIRU Hedges Template. http://hiru.mcmaster.ca/hiru/HIRU_Hedges_home.aspx. Accessed August 11, 2008.

17. Spitzer WO, Feinstein AR, Sackett DL. What is a health care trial? *JAMA.*1975;233:161-163.

18. Jenkins J, Hubbard S. History of clinical trials. *Semin Oncol Nurs.* 1991;7:228-234.

19. Grimes DA. Clinical research in ancient Babylon: methodologic insights from the book of Daniel. *Obstet Gynecol.* 1995;86:1031-1034.

20. Diehl HS, Baker AB, Cowan AD. Cold vaccines: an evaluation based on a control study. *JAMA.*1938;111:1168-1173.

21. Streptomycin treatment of tuberculosis. *Br Med J.* 1948;2:769-782.

22. Doll R, Hill AB. Smoking and carcinoma of the lung; preliminary report. *Br Med J.* 1950;2:739-748.

23. Pearson K. Report on certain enteric fever inoculation statistics. *Br Med J.*1904;3:1243-1246.

24. Kinsey VE. Retrolental fibroplasia; cooperative study of retrolental fibroplasia and the use of oxygen. *AMA Arch Ophthalmol.* 1956;56:481-543.

25. MacArthur AC, Le ND, Abanto ZU, Gallagher RP. Occupational female breast and reproductive cancer mortality in British Columbia, Canada, 1950-94. *Occup Med (Lond).* 2007 Jun;57(4):246-253.

2

Therapy, Prevention and Control, and Quality Improvement

Ann McKibbon

INTRODUCTION

Therapy is the most common category of research methodology. Therapy studies provide evidence that some aspect of care is better than another (e.g., a new drug) or at least equivalent to current care with some increased benefits (e.g., minimally invasive surgery that shortens hospital stay). Physicians refer to these studies as **therapy or treatment**, while nurses use the term **interventions**. The main methodology is a randomized controlled trial, which will be the main focus of this chapter. Issues of prevention--such as keeping something like asthma from developing for the first time (primary prevention) or from recurring (secondary prevention)--are also studied using randomized controlled trial methodologies, as are quality improvement studies. Quality improvement refers to issues of improving the care process often using education, changes in the process of care (e.g., adding a nurse to a ward to optimize the care process or instituting a stroke unit in a hospital), or adding information technology to aid clinical decision making (e.g., a clinical decision support system to guide the choice of medications or a reminder system to improve the rate of immunization for infants). We start this chapter, as we do with all chapters, using a study that illustrates the issues important to understanding the category of research we are considering.

CLINICAL EXAMPLE

Leg ulcers are a substantial problem for many people although the burden of care is greater for seniors and their care providers. Ulcers or wounds can be acute as in a surgical incision or traffic accident or chronic. Certain populations, such as the elderly and those with diabetes, often have ulcers or wounds that last a substantial length of time and prone to return. Healing often takes 4 to 6 weeks. Considerable care is needed in both outpatient and inpatient settings to speed healing and prevent spread. In the past decade, honey has gained considerable attention in relation to its perceived benefits in wound healing. Used in healing for more than 4500 years, the Egyptians left the earliest evidence of honey for wound healing. Moore and colleagues[1] collected 7 randomized controlled trials on honey and wound healing and combined the findings from these trials (see Chapter 10). This summary showed that for acute wounds such as burns, honey may have healing potential. No data, however, are available for chronic wounds. Therefore, Jull and colleagues,[2] who are involved in treating leg ulcers, obtained funding from the Health Research Council of New Zealand to study if honey-impregnated dressings were more effective than usual care (bandaging of choice by health care professionals). The investigators of the study chose their outcome to be the rate of complete healing at 12 weeks.

Jull and colleagues calculated that if they studied 400 participants with chronic leg ulcers they would be able to determine if the honey bandages were more effective (this is called sample size determination). From May 2004 until September 2005, they asked 392 people with leg ulcers if they wanted to be part of the study. Of these, 368 agreed and were included. After determining if each person were eligible according to the study inclusion and exclusion criteria, the study nurse called the central randomization center. Study personnel at this center recorded the participant's name and other information related to the study. They then provided a random allocation so that the participant received leg ulcer care using either the honey-impregnated bandages (study group) or usual care with the type of bandages chosen by the clinician looking after that patient (control group).

The study group (honey) had 187 patients and the control group (usual bandages) had 181 patients. After 12 weeks of receiving their allocated care, the participants were assessed to determine if the leg ulcers were healed (main outcome measure) as well as the time taken to heal, size of unhealed ulcers, infections in the wounds, and other adverse effects. All participants who started the trial were included in the final analyses despite the fact that some stopped using the honey dressings and 2 people had moved and could not be traced. Those who died or were not available for assessment were assumed to have an unhealed ulcer in these final analyses.

Jull and colleagues entered into the study postulating that after 12 weeks more ulcers in the honey-dressing group would be healed and that their healing would be faster. The investigators based this assumption on results from similar studies in other types of wounds. They were disappointed, however. The number and proportion of healed wounds was substantially the same (although a tiny bit higher in the honey group). The honey group had 104 healed ulcers (55.6%) and the control group had 90 healed ulcers (49.7%). Time to healing was also similar in the 2 groups (63.5 days in the honey-dressing group vs. 65.3 days in the usual-care group). No differences were found for quality of life (measured with questionnaires) and costs to the health care system. The only differences found between the groups were that more adverse effects such as pain were found in the honey-dressing group. The investigators concluded that, based on their results, honey-impregnated bandages are not more effective for healing leg ulcers than existing methods.

HOW THERAPY TRIALS ARE DONE

A rigorous or well-done therapy trial starts with a group of persons, all of whom have the disease or condition that is to be studied if the trial is designed to treat the condition. Alternately all participants are free of the condition to be studied if the intent is to study how best to prevent it from occurring (prevention study). Because the goal is to determine if a treatment or regimen is better, or at least as good as, another process or intervention, multiple groups are needed so that this comparison can be made. Two or more interventions or treatments are compared in a single study population. To make this comparison as true and replicable as possible, patients are divided into two or more groups that should be as equivalent as possible, so that at the end of the study, any differences seen can be attributed to the interventions. To get similar groups, the participants should be placed into groups using an unbiased allocation method. Patients in each group take their allotted therapy (drug, surgery, honey-impregnated bandages, music, placebo, and so on). After a specified period, researchers measure all outcomes of interest in all participants and compare the group results, looking for differences that can be attributed to the treatments. Again, for a true comparison, these study groups must be as similar as possible in all respects *except for the treatment or other intervention such as education.*

The study design, or methodology, used for evaluating therapeutic, prevention, or quality improvement interventions is called a **randomized controlled trial** or a **controlled clinical trial**. An example of a *therapy trial* is whether amoxicillin is better than placebo to cure otitis media. An example of a *prevention study* would be assertiveness training workshops combined with follow-up sessions and peer counseling at the start of each high school semester for teenaged boys and girls to reduce the rates of pregnancy and sexually transmitted diseases in the following semesters. An example of a *quality improvement* trial is adding routine notes to the charts of ambulatory patients reminding clinicians of the need for women to be screened for breast cancer; another is implementing case managers in hospital wards to improve the care process as well as patient outcomes of increased satisfaction, shorter hospital stays, and lower infection rates after surgery.

COMPARATIVE GROUPS

To be sure that the groups are as similar as possible at the start of the study, patients are put into each study group using an allocation method that is unbiased (no personal preference on anyone's part should influence group assignment). Two research methods issues come into play here: allocation concealment and random allocation.

Allocation Concealment

Allocation concealment happens during enrollment of the participants into the study. After being told about the study, participants often form preferences for being in 1 group or another. Health professionals may also want a certain patient to be in a specific group. To keep preferences from consciously or unconsciously influencing group allocation, several processes can be put in place that avoid bias or make for unequal study groups at baseline. Two of the most common are:

- Opaque, sequentially numbered, sealed envelopes containing the next group assignment. Once the patient has consented and baseline information is obtained, the study staff member will open the envelope to ascertain the group assignment.
- Telephone or internet services that collect patient information after consent and then provide the next allocation.

Jull et al[2] used the telephone method to ensure allocation concealment for the honey-bandage study.

Random Allocation

Random allocation deals with how the groups are formed. Ideally, study participants should have the same probability of going into each group. To perform the allocation, researchers use such techniques as random number tables, coin tosses, or other, similar methods to set up allocation sequences for patients. This can be done before the study starts or during the study itself. Allocation to study groups by birth date (odd vs even or first half of the year or month vs second half), patient chart number (odd vs even), or day of week seen in the clinic is not random. These methods are, however, better than clinician or patient preference to ensure comparability of groups.

Randomization can be done with "parts" of people. For example, half of one's head washed with shampoo A and half with shampoo B to assess comparative abilities of the products to kill head lice and their eggs, or arms randomly allocated to intravenous insertion of a catheter using the standard landmark guidance procedure or ultrasonography. Most often persons are allocated, but towns, wards, schools, hospitals, bus stops, and so on have been allocated in well-designed studies. The research question and outcomes dictate the unit randomized.

Groups do not need to be the same size. Often the sizes are similar, but randomization does not guarantee exactly equal numbers. Indeed, some studies purposely involve unequal numbers in each group. For example, Maizels et al[3] studied intranasal lidocaine compared with placebo for migraine pain relief. Twice as many people (58:28) were allocated to receive the intranasal lidocaine as were allocated to receive placebo (intranasal saline solution). These unequal groups were formed because of ethical and common sense issues of withholding medication from persons with migraine headache pain. The analyses at the end of the study can factor and adjust for the difference in group size.

BLINDING

In addition to the random allocation in therapy trials, patients, health care workers, and study personnel should not know, if feasible, the group to which the patient is assigned. This is called blinding or masking and it avoids what is commonly called measurement bias. Human nature being what it is, the expectations of patients, health care workers, and researchers are strong and can unconsciously influence the experience and reporting of outcomes. Quite often, with the best of intentions, people report what they think should be happening or what they expect others to think should be happening. To minimize these potentially biased perceptions, neither the health care worker nor the patient should know which group he or she is in, that is, what treatment a patient is receiving. As an example of how expectations rather then actual events affect outcomes, an early vitamin C study was funded by the U.S. National Institutes of Health and the results were published in 1975.[4] This trial was designed and funded to definitively prove what researchers had reported since 1938: that vitamin C was the wonder drug to prevent and cure the common cold. After enrollment, people were randomly given either vitamin C or powdered sucrose in similar capsules, and instructed to take them on the same, fixed schedule. They were to report all colds and related symptoms. Some study participants, knowing the taste difference between the vitamin C and sugar, opened the capsules and tasted them. (This is known as **code breaking**.)

When people reported their outcomes in the vitamin C study (i.e., cold symptoms) they also told the researchers that they had "broken the code." Knowing that some persons had discovered to which group they had been assigned, the researchers analyzed these additional data to compare rates of cold symptoms in the persons who knew what they were taking and in the persons who did not know—called a **subgroup analysis**. The rates of colds and symptoms did not differ in these 2 subgroups, indicating that the code breaking had probably not affected the results. Controversy continues, however, around the results of the study and around questions of proper data analysis, assessment of other biases, code breaking, and trial methods, and researchers are still not confident they have completely evaluated whether vitamin C prevents or reduces the burden of the common cold.

Adequate blinding takes much planning, preparation, and creativity by the researchers designing the methods. In a study comparing 2 drug treatments for lowering cholesterol, 1 drug needed to be taken once a day at bedtime. The other drug was taken 3 times a day at meals. Each person in the trial took 4 pills a day: 1 with each meal and 1 at bedtime. Some of the pills were placebos and some were "real" medicine. Texture, taste, color, and other features were closely matched for placebo and active medicine.

Some studies have gone to extremes to incorporate blinding. One surgery trial many years ago randomized patients to surgery or no surgery after the patients had gone to the operating room, been prepped and anesthetized, and the operation started. When the patients were ready for the surgery to start, the surgeon received notification of the random allocation. Half the patients had surgery and the other half did not. For the people not randomized to the surgery group, the surgery was terminated and they were returned to their rooms to be given the alternate treatment—in this case medication. Although creative, this type of blinding would likely not be done today because of ethical concerns and the growing awareness of patients' rights and the obligations of researchers to make full disclosure of information about the total trial to the participants before they agree to join the study.

Use of a placebo can present problems, or benefits. The placebo effect happens when people feel that their treatment is "real" and they "improve." Approximately 35% to 75% of patients who get placebo medication or treatment report improvements in their conditions.[5] The most dramatic example of this placebo effect is a study by Moseley et al.[6] They took 180 people with osteoarthritis of the knee and randomized people to surgery (arthroscopic debridement), less intensive surgery (arthroscopic lavage), or placebo surgery. All patients were anesthetized and were given identical skin portals—cuts that allowed entry of the surgical tools. After 2 years, no differences were seen for patient satisfaction or any clinical outcomes when the 3 groups were compared. The placebo effect was as strong as real surgery. Alternately it could be said that surgery was not better than placebo for improving satisfaction or outcomes.

Single-, Double-, and Triple-Blinding

Several groups of persons are often involved in health care studies and each can be blinded to the study groups:

- Patients or participants who are being studied in the trial as well as their informal caregivers
- Their health professionals (nurses and physicians)
- Study personnel who interact with the study participants

- Outcome assessors who assess the final state of the participants at the end of the trial
- Data analysts and those that prepare the final reports and manuscripts
- Funding providers

Single blinding refers to a study when 1 group only is blinded to the intervention. Often it is either the patient *or* the health professional who does not know the study allocation. **Double-blinding** refers to 2 groups blinded to the intervention, usually the health professional *and* the patient both do not know which medicine or study intervention the patient is receiving. **Triple-blinding** means that 3 groups do not know which treatment is active therapy and which is placebo or standard therapy until final data analysis is complete. Multiple blinding is especially important for trials sponsored by commercial groups, including drug companies. The companies are often criticized for putting their concern for profits above reporting negative trials of their products. Full-scale blinding helps all users of health care research have confidence in the final published results. Double-blinding is the most common form of blinding reported, although no consensus exists as to which groups are blinded.

Blinding Is Not Always Possible

In some cases, it is not possible to blind a study because of logistical or ethical problems. For example, heart surgeons undertook surgery on both warm and cooled hearts in a surgery study in Toronto.[7] Historically, surgeons thought chilled hearts needed less oxygen, and therefore suffered less tissue damage during operations than hearts that were kept at body temperature during surgery. Researchers disputed this, and a randomized controlled trial was done to determine whether this assumption of cold hearts accruing less damage during surgery was true. Because it was not possible to blind the surgeons to the temperature of the hearts on which they operated, the researchers did not even try. Instead, they put their energies into making sure the outcomes measured (death, morbidity, time off work, and so on) were assessed in as unbiased a way as possible. To do this, neither the patients nor the persons who assessed the outcomes knew the procedure each patient received, and the surgeons were not involved in assessing any of the study outcomes related to the patients. At the end of the study patients whose hearts were chilled had worse outcomes. Chilling of hearts during cardiac surgery is no longer done.

Another example where blinding could not take place is a study of premature babies. Newborn babies, especially premature ones, do not regulate their internal temperatures well. It is important for the babies' wellbeing to keep their body temperature within a normal range. A randomized controlled trial was undertaken in which babies were assigned to either higher thermostat settings on their isolets, or to wearing hats.[8] The theoretical basis of the study was that most body heat is lost through the head. During the interim and final study assessments of the infants, the babies were not wearing hats. They were also assessed by a study staff member who had no knowledge of each infant's hat status during the stay in the neonatal intensive care unit. The higher thermostat settings did more harm than good, and babies in most neonatal intensive care units now wear hats.

Ophthalmologists and "Masked" Studies

Blinding also goes by other names. For example, ophthalmologists who deal with patients with vision problems prefer the term **masked**. Gwon studied topical ofloxacin compared with gentamicin for treatment of internal ocular infection[9] and reported the blinding of the study using the term "masked." **Sham**, **dummy**, and **double dummy** are other terms that refer to placebos and blinding. These terms are used more often in European studies than in studies conducted in North America.

FOLLOW-UP

Participant follow-up is also very important in understanding, evaluating, and applying randomized controlled trial results. Follow-up deals with the ability of the study personnel to account for all of the patients who enter the study. People may lose interest or move and it becomes difficult to find all of a study's participants. Most methodologists insist that at least 80% of all participants who were randomized at the start of the study be analyzed at the end of the study for the results to be valid or "true." This means accounting for all participants who withdrew from the treatments (keeping this number to a minimum), dropped out, or were otherwise lost. If more than 20% of the participants were lost because they became much better, or much worse, with specific treatments, the study's results might not be generalizable, i.e., not applicable to others outside the study. (**Generalizability** is the degree to which the results can be taken from a specific research study and applied to other groups of persons—steps 3 and 4 in the 5 step EBHC process; see Chapter 1.)

Attaining good follow-up can be easier or harder, depending on the study. An example of easy follow-up is a short-term study designed to assess the relative benefits of standard-dose intravenous pain relief with a patient-controlled arrangement using a pump injection system within the first 24 hours of cardiac surgery. Such a study would easily have a 100% follow-up rate. Follow-up is much more difficult when the study lasts longer, the patients are more mobile, and few incentives exist to keep patients interested. Examples of difficult follow-up would be a program to cure and prevent the spread of tuberculosis in homeless persons, methadone and counseling studies over a period of years in persons with substance abuse problems, and drug trials where the medications have major side effects with few obvious favorable outcomes as seen in some cholesterol-lowering agents.

UNDERSTANDING THERAPY STATISTICS

In addition to understanding how a therapy trial is done and how it is indexed and reported, anyone interested in health care or EBHC needs to know the common conventions authors use to report study outcomes. The following is a simple nonclinical example to start our discussions.

Assume that the health care budget cuts are too difficult and frustrating, and you have decided that, instead of your present job, you want to start a cream cheese factory and produce a good-tasting, low-fat product. After several months of work, your product tastes wonderful, and production costs and uptake by your market seem to suggest your endeavors will be cost effective. Marketing is your next step in getting the cheese on the grocery shelves. You tentatively pick the name "Litee-Bitees." The marketing company feels that the taste is not enough for product success and urges you to move to presenting your product in terms of numbers. Here is what you start with:

- The "other brand" cream cheese has a 40% butterfat content
- Your low-fat Litee-Bitees has a 20% butterfat content

How are you going to best describe and advertise your product using these numbers?

You can describe the difference in fat content in the following ways:

- Your cream cheese has 20% less than theirs; or
- Theirs has 20% more butterfat than yours.

These 2 figures represent an *absolute* difference (e.g., from 40% to 20% is a 20% reduction, or from 20% to 40% is a 20% increase in butterfat).

We can also look at the difference in numbers (percentages of butter fat) from a relative point of view. We can express the difference in fat content by saying that, taking into account the baseline (i.e., ours at 20% and theirs at 40%):

- Yours has a 50% reduction in fat levels compared with theirs; or
- Theirs has a 100% increase in fat levels compared with yours.

These two statistics or figures represent a *relative* difference. For example, starting at 40% and going to 20% cuts the fat in half—a 50% reduction, and going from 20 to 40% doubles the fat—a 100% increase. Both the 2 absolute differences (20%) and the 2 relative differences (50% and 100%) are correct representations of the differences in fat levels between the 2 brands of cream cheese.

Like you and your cream cheese, clinicians have many ways of describing the results of clinical trials: even more than the absolute and relative differences seen in the cream cheese example. Frick et al[10] studied patients who had high levels of cholesterol. They wanted to lower the cholesterol levels and prevent myocardial infarction using the drug gemfibrozil. After 5 years they found that, for patients who had received placebo, 3.9% of the persons had had a myocardial infarction. For patients who had received gemfibrozil, the rate of myocardial infarction was 2.3%. The differences between, and the clinical implications, of the 3.9% and 2.3% results can be represented by any of the following 7 statistics (the name of the statistic is in parentheses after the statistic itself):

- 1.6% fewer patients had myocardial infarctions (**absolute risk reduction**).
- 41% reduction in the rate of myocardial infarction (**relative risk reduction**).
- A clinician would need to treat 71 patients for 5 years to prevent 1 additional patient from having a myocardial infarction (**number needed to treat**).
- 389,000 pills would have to be taken to prevent 1 additional patient from having a myocardial infarction (**number of pills needed to be taken**).
- Each patient treated increased his/her time with no myocardial infarction on average by 15 weeks (**disease-free survival**).
- Each life-year saved cost U.S. $47,523 (**life-year cost savings**).
- Gemfibrozil is better than placebo ($P < .01$) (**P-value** comparison).

Hux and Naylor[11] gave 100 people most of the above numbers and asked them to choose if they would take the study drug based on their perceptions of the accompanying numbers. Their responses and some explanation of the figures are summarized below.

- The **absolute risk reduction** is 1.6% fewer deaths—the arithmetic difference between 3.9% and 2.3%. It is the simplest statistic. This absolute risk reduction is calculated as the difference in rates (3.9% – 2.3% = 1.6%). Forty-two percent of the participants in the survey by Hux and Naylor would choose to take gemfibrozil if they were given the absolute risk reduction numbers. This 1.6% number and calculation are conceptually identical to the 20% differences in the cream cheese example.
- The **relative risk reduction** is a 41% reduction—conceptually identical to the 50% and 100% calculated in the cream cheese example. This is calculated as the difference (1.6%) divided by the rate in the placebo group as a percentage 1.6/3.9 = 0.41 or 41%. Even though the relative risk reduction is derived from the same data, 88% of the Hux and Naylor participants would choose to take gemfibrozil when given this relative risk reduction statistic—almost double the number of people who state they would take it based on absolute differences.

- The **number (of persons) needed-to-treat (NNT)** is 63 to prevent 1 additional myocardial infarction at 5 years. Another way of putting this is that for every 63 patients who received gemfibrozil for 5 years, 1 additional myocardial infarction would be prevented. The NNT number is calculated by the formula

$$100\%/\text{Absolute difference} = 100/1.6 = 63$$

  Thirty-one percent of the Hux and Naylor participants would choose to take the drug given the NNT figures—far fewer than the first 2 numbers given (absolute and relative risk reductions).

- The **disease-free survival** time is 15 weeks, and 40% of the Hux and Naylor participants would choose to take the drug based on these results.

Hux and Naylor did not give the **cost-per-life-year-saved** data, **the number of pills needed to be taken** to prevent 1 additional event, or the P-**value** to the participants for assessment. *P*-values are a measure of the probability of obtaining the same observed difference between the groups or a larger difference if the trial were repeated using the same people. The smaller the *P*-value, the more likely the observed difference did not occur by chance alone but by "true" differences in the groups—hopefully related to the treatments that were randomized. By convention, if the *P*-value is less than 0.05 (or 5%) one can start to "believe" the results. The *P*-values on their own are even less helpful than some of the other numbers researchers use to present their results of their studies. Differences in risk between study groups are most often represented as absolute differences and relative differences, with the numbers needed-to-treat data becoming more common over time. You have already seen absolute and relative differences in the cream cheese example.

Therapy articles report various statistics to show the magnitude and direction of the differences between the study groups. We will discuss some of the more widely used statistics in the next several sections and then present some of the lesser used statistics. Statistics are just a numerical language used to describe what has happened to the people involved at the end of a trial or study and the observed differences, if present, across the groups.

Trials are designed in 1 of 2 "directions." They are most often designed to study if we can prevent "bad" things from happening or to lessen the effects of the bad things. These bad things are often such things as death, depression, pain, loneliness, high cholesterol levels, and so on. When studies are designed to reduce the occurrence of these bad things, we talk about the "risk" for the bad event and consequently work to reduce the risk. For example, Weintraub and colleagues[12] instituted a team sports program for children in a low income, racially mixed ethnic community. This randomized controlled trial sought to decrease the occurrence or rate of high body mass index in young children through an after school soccer program. Similarly Gaede and colleagues[13] showed that a multifactorial intervention with intensive targeted care goals and behavior modification for middle-aged patients with diabetes reduced the risk for or occurrence of death, or the progression of their diabetes compared with patients who received standard intensive care.

Some studies are designed to increase the occurrence of "good" things, such as improved depression scores, better quality of life, increased wages, greater self-assurance scores, and longer walking distances. These increases in good things are referred to as "benefit" increases. In the trial of personalized parent-voice smoke alarms, Smith and colleagues[14] showed that children who were asleep woke more quickly and more often, and exited their rooms faster than if the smoke alarm emitted the standard tones. It is a good thing to awaken children and speed their exits when a smoke detector is activated. Both good and bad things can be combined in the same trial also. Weintraub and colleagues[12] also sought to increase the amount of physical activity in children in their after-school soccer program.

Absolute Risk or Benefit Difference

The absolute difference is the arithmetic difference between the rates of events in the intervention, or the experimental group and the control group. This difference can be expressed in 4 different ways, depending on what outcome is being measured (whether "good" or "bad"), and whether the rates of the outcome events are increased or decreased when comparing the study groups:

- An **absolute risk reduction** occurs when the risk of a bad event (e.g., death, fever, myocardial infarction, or recurrence) decreases as a result of an intervention, compared with control treatment or no treatment. (This is a desirable situation.)
- An **absolute benefit increase** occurs when the risk of a good event (e.g., abstinence from alcohol, successful pregnancy, exercise time, or base salary) increases when an intervention is compared with control treatment or no treatment. (This again, is a desirable situation.)
- An **absolute risk increase** occurs when the risk of a bad event (e.g., breast cancer after hormone replacement therapy or gastrointestinal hemorrhage after taking aspirin to prevent strokes) increases when an intervention is compared with control treatment or no treatment. (This is not a desirable situation but it can occur in studies.)
- An **absolute benefit reduction** occurs when the benefit of a good outcome decreases (e.g., teaching reading skills with whole language techniques did not produce more or better readers by 5th grade—the control group did better than the experimental or intervention group). (This is not good, of course.)

Relative Risk or Benefit Difference

The **relative risk or benefit difference** is the proportional difference between the rates of events in the experimental group and the control group, taking into account the control group rate (i.e., the rate that would have occurred without the intervention drug or program). Relative differences are always bigger than absolute differences, and often tend to inflate perceptions of what the results of the study truly are. Recall the cream cheese example with a 20% absolute difference between your and other products and a 50% increase or 100% relative difference. Some clinicians admit using relative numbers (the larger numbers) in describing a treatment choice when they want to encourage the patient to choose the treatment, and using absolute numbers (the smaller numbers) when they would like the patients not to choose the treatment.

The relative risk difference is calculated by dividing the absolute difference by the control rate; that is:

(Experimental or intervention rate – Control rate)/Control rate

It can be expressed similarly to the above in that 4 things can happen:

- Relative risk reduction
- Relative benefit increase
- Relative risk increase
- Relative benefit reduction

Number Needed-to-Treat

The **number needed-to-treat (NNT)** is defined as the number of patients that a clinician would need to treat with the experimental treatment or intervention to achieve 1 additional patient who has a favorable response or outcome. NNT is one of the best methods for comparing how big the effects of a new treatment or therapy would be. The smaller the NNT––that is, the fewer patients one would need to treat to see 1 additional benefit happen or 1 risk be avoided––the better it is for patients and the health care system. As an example of a small NNT, the NNT for a new anti-nausea drug for children during chemotherapy is 3.[15] This means that 3 children would have to be treated with the drug to have 1 additional child be protected from being nauseous after chemotherapy compared with what would have happened if the children had not been treated for nausea during chemotherapy. Another example showing a much larger value is an NNT of approximately 5900 per year to save 1 life by testing adults to determine if they have colorectal cancer by using fecal occult blood screening.[16] This means that 5900 persons would need to be screened for colorectal cancer to prevent 1 additional death at 1 year. In summary, the smaller the NNT, the more effective is the treatment. Although NNT is not that easy to understand at first glance, it is a representation of the results of studies that is being used more frequently.

The NNT is calculated as 100/absolute difference, and can be either "number needed-to-treat" for studies with results that show that the new treatment is helpful or "number needed-to harm" (NNH) for studies where the results are in the opposite direction—the new treatment is actually harmful compared with standard care. For example, an NNH of 42 would mean that, for every 42 persons with rheumatoid arthritis who were treated with nonsteroidal anti-inflammatory agents, 1 additional person would have a major gastrointestinal hemorrhage within 2 years.

Confidence Intervals and *P*-Values

The **confidence interval (CI)** quantifies the uncertainty of a result or statistic. A 95% CI represents the range of values within which we can be 95% sure that the number or result given falls within that range if we repeated the study. For example, a weight loss study might find that the mean difference in weight loss in the 2 groups was 5 kg with a 95% CI of $\pm$ 2 kg. Representation of this would be in the form 5 kg, 95% CI 3 to 7. This means that if we repeated the study 100 times, the mean difference in weight loss between the groups would be between 3 and 7 kg for 95 of the trials. Because these 95 hypothetical trials have an outcome of weight loss between 3 and 7 kg, we say that this result is statistically significant—we are confident that this weight loss program is effective and we can recommend it to patients once we assess that the problems or costs of the program are reasonable and participants would accept them.

Sometimes confidence intervals are mistaken for standard deviation (SD) data. Standard deviations measure the "spread" of the data. Calculation of SDs can be a bit tedious. The SD for the above weight loss example is presented in the form 5 $\pm$ 2 kg. By definition the $\pm$ value (in this case 4 kg with 2 being above 5 and 2 being below) indicates that approximately 66% of the participants obtained values between these 2 data points—that is, two-thirds of the people in the study lost between 3 and 7 pounds. Careful reading is often needed to determine if authors are providing 95% CI or SD data.

Another way of measuring the statistical significance (or surety) of a trial is to use a *P*-value. *P*-values are associated with the probability of getting the result demonstrated in a study or a result that is more extreme by chance alone. Taking this definition and applying it to study results, if you have a study that says that exercise is better than drug A for increasing walking distances in elderly people with a *P*-value of 0.05, you are going to be correct in your assumption of the value of exercise at least 95% of the time. As the *P*-value gets smaller, you become more "sure" of the results. CIs are more informative than *P*-values as they give an idea of the magnitude of the uncertainty/certainty rather than just a statement about its probability. A general rule of thumb is that CIs should be narrow and the

P-values small for you to be relatively sure of the results and their potential for applicability.

Calculations

One of the best ways to understand numerical presentations of data is to actually do the calculations oneself. The following data come from Smith et al[14] and their study of smoke alarms that use standard tones (usual situation) compared with a potential innovation (the voice of the child's mother urging the child to wake and leave the bedroom because of fire or smoke). The relevant numbers follow.

The study enrolled 24 healthy children between the ages of 6 and 12 years. Their parents worked at the Columbus Children's Hospital and the children received their primary health care at that center. The main outcome of the study was whether the child awoke after hearing the alarm with standard tones and the mother's voice. This study assessed the children "twice" in the process of testing both of the alarm systems. At the start of the study the children were trained how to perform a "self-rescue escape procedure" when they heard either alarm while asleep. The children were observed in a sleep laboratory and once asleep were allocated to hear the standard tone alarm or their mother's voice alarm in random order. The children were considered to be both "controls" and intervention participants. At the end of the study

- 23 of 24 children (96%) awoke after hearing the alarm with their mother's voice
- 14 of 24 children (58%) awoke after hearing the alarm with standard tones

The first step in working with the numbers in the study is to decide if the outcome is "good" or "bad." In this case, being awoken and accomplishing a safe quick exit, even in a simulated situation, is good. (We are also looking at the *proportion* of people with outcomes. If we were looking at outcomes such as average weight loss in a diet study we would be using other methods of analyzing the results.) Therefore, we are looking at benefits and not risks (or harms). Because many more children (a higher proportion) woke after hearing their mother's voice, we will be calculating benefit increases as a result of the voice alarm. Please fill in the blanks. Suggested correct answers follow.

Rate of waking with standard alarm (control)	58%
Rate of waking with mother's voice (experimental)	96%

Absolute Benefit

Reduction? Increase?

Control rate – Experimental rate

_____ – _____

= _____

Relative Risk

Reduction? Increase?

(Control rate – Experimental rate)/Control rate

(_____ – _____)/(_____)

= _____ / _____

= _____

Number Needed-to-Treat

100/(Control rate – Experimental rate)

= 100/(_____)

= _____

Absolute Benefit

Increase

Control rate – Experimental rate

$\underline{\quad 58\% \quad}$ – $\underline{\quad 96\% \quad}$

= 38%

Putting this into words, the alarm using the mother's voice lead to an absolute benefit increase of 38% compared with standard tone alarms.

Relative Benefit

Increase

(Control rate – Experimental rate)/Control rate

$\underline{\quad (96\% \quad}$ – $\underline{\quad 58\%) \quad}$ / $\underline{\quad (58\%) \quad}$

= $\underline{\quad 38\% \quad}$ / $\underline{\quad 58\% \quad}$

= $\underline{\quad 66\% \quad}$

The relative benefit of using a mother's voice in a fire alarm was 66% compared with standard tone alarms.

Number Needed-to-Treat

100/(Control rate – Experimental rate)

= 100 / ($\underline{\quad 38 \quad}$)

= $\underline{\quad 2.6 \quad}$

= $\underline{\quad 3 \quad}$

Standard procedure using NNTs is to always round **up** to the next whole number as we do not treat parts of people. Therefore, the NNT with a smoke alarm that uses the mother's voice is 3 to encounter 1 additional child exiting a room safely after being awoken by the alarm. This is a very small number. This study was published in 2006 and one wonders why we have not moved to implementing a mother's voice in all smoke detectors. Approximately 4000 children die in their beds from fires and smoke annually[14] in the United States and all countries encounter similar rates of fire and smoke deaths. This link provides a sample of a parent's recorded voice for one commercial product(http://www.smarthome.com/audio/7563.wav).

SUMMARY

Therapy, prevention and control, and quality improvement studies use a randomized controlled trial study design. Important aspects of the studies are allocation, concealment, randomization, blinding, and follow-up. A fuller description of clinical trials is included in many publications including a *BMJ* book by Jadad.[17] The Evidence Based Medicine Working Group[18] lists the following issues as important to understanding and evaluation RCTs:

- The intervention and the control groups started with the same prognosis at the beginning of the trial
- Randomization of the participants or patients to study groups
- Allocation is concealed to all those involved in the trial who may have influence on which group a person might be assigned
- Patients have the same prognostic factors at the start of the trial
- Patients maintained the prognostic balance throughout the trial and at the end
- Blinding done when possible and other measures used to protect the study from bias if blinding presented challenges
- Patients analyzed according to the group to which they were allocated
- The trial was not stopped early except for extremely good reasons
- The magnitude of the treatment effect and the direction is given
- Precision of the treatment effects is provided
- Outcomes of interest were evaluated
- Consideration if the benefits are worth the potential harms and costs

SEARCHING METHODOLOGY

The next section in this chapter examines how indexers who produce the 4 large electronic databases index for the study methodology. Both index terms and the terms and phrases authors use in their titles and abstracts (called **textwords**) can be used to construct search strategies. After the tables for MEDLINE, CINAHL, PsycINFO, and EMBASE/Excerpta Medica, several examples of research studies are included, with indexing and textwords related to methodology highlighted. Examining the indexing and author use of methods terms can help us understand how best to retrieve randomized controlled trials from the literature.

MEDLINE

MeSH, Subheadings, Publication Types, and Textwords

MeSH (Medical Subject Headings — Index Terms)

Placebos*

"Outcome and process assessment (health care)" (can be exploded)
"Outcome assessment (health care)" (can be exploded)
"Process assessment (health care)"
"Sensitivity and specificity"
"Sensitivity and specificity" (can be exploded)
Animal use alternatives (can be exploded)
Clinical protocols
Clinical trials as topic (can be exploded)
Clinical trials as topic, phase i
Clinical trials as topic, phase ii
Clinical trials as topic, phase iii
Clinical trials as topic, phase iv
Comparative study
Confidence intervals
Controlled clinical trials (can be exploded)
Cross-over studies
Disease-free survival
Double-blind method
Epidemiologic research design (can be exploded)
Evaluation studies (can be exploded)
Feasibility studies
Follow-up studies
Human genome project
Intervention studies
Logistic models
Longitudinal studies (can be exploded)
Matched-pair analysis
Medical futility
Meta-analysis
Multicenter studies
Observation
Odds ratio
Patient selection
Peer review, research

---

*Indicates a preferred term as determined in the Clinical Hedges Study.[20,21]

Pilot projects
Proportional hazards models
Prospective studies
Random allocation
Randomized controlled trials
Regression analysis (can be exploded)
Reproducibility of results
Research (can be exploded)
Research design (can be exploded)
Risk (can be exploded)
Risk adjustment
Risk assessment (can be exploded)
Risk factors
Sample size
Sampling studies
Single-blind method
Survival analysis (can be exploded)
Treatment failure
Treatment outcome (can be exploded)

Subheadings

Therapeutic use* (can be exploded)

Adverse effects (can be exploded)
Chemically induced
Contraindications
Diet therapy
Drug therapy
Nursing
Psychology
Prevention and control
Radiotherapy
Rehabilitation
Surgery (can be exploded)
Therapy (can be exploded)

Publication Types

Clinical trial*
Randomized controlled trial*

Clinical trial, phase i

---

*Indicates a preferred term as determined in the Clinical Hedges Study.[20,21]

Clinical trial, phase ii
Clinical trial, phase iii
Clinical trial, phase iv
Controlled clinical trial
Evaluation studies
Multicenter study
Validation studies

Textwords (Same List Is Used for All 4 Databases)

Clinical trial:*
Contrast*
Double-blind*
Random assigned*

Random:
Randomized:
Absolute benefit increas:
Absolute benefit reduct:
Absolute risk differenc:
Absolute risk increas:
Absolute risk reduct:
Adverse effect:
Advers: effect:
Allocation conceal:
Blinded
Central random:
Centrally random:
Clinical stud:
Comparative clinical stud:
Comparative clinical trial:
Comparative stud:
Comparative trial:
Concealed allocation
Confidence interval:
CI
Controlled clinical stud:
Controlled clinical trial:
Controlled stud:
Control: stud:
Controlled trial:
Control: trial:
Crossover procedure:

---

*Indicates a preferred term as determined in the Clinical Hedges Study.[20-24]

Cross-over procedure:
Crossover stud:
Cross-over stud:
Crossover trial:
Cross-over trial:
Double-dummy
Double mask:
Effectiveness
Effectiveness stud:
Effectiveness trial:
Efficacy
Efficacy analys:
Efficacy stud:
Efficacy trial:
Experiment:
Experimental stud:
Experimental trial:
Factorial design:
Feasibility stud:
Feasibility trial:
Followup stud:
Follow-up stud:
Followup trial:
Follow-up trial:
Hazard ratio:
HR
Intention to treat
Intention to treat analys:
Intervention stud:
Intervention trial:
Longitudinal stud:
Longitudinal trial:
Mask:
Multicenter stud:
Multicentre stud:
Multicenter trial:
Multicentre trial:
Number needed to harm
Numbers needed to harm
Number needed to treat
Numbers needed to treat
NNT
NNH
Odds ratio

OR
Outcome assessment:
Per protocol
Per protocol analys:
Phase 2
Phase 3
Phase 4
Phase ii
Phase iii
Phase iv
Pilot stud:
Pilot trial:
Placebo:
Prevention stud:
Prevention trial:
Prospective stud:
Prospective trial:
Quadruple-blind:
Quadruple mask:
Random allocation
Random: allocation
Random assignment
Random: assignment
Randomised clinical stud:
Randomized clinical stud:
Random: clinical stud:
Randomised clinical trial:
Randomized clinical trial:
Random: clinical trial:
Randomised controlled stud:
Randomized controlled stud:
Random: controlled stud:
Randomised controlled trial:
Randomized controlled trial:
Random: controlled trial:
Randomised control stud:
Randomized control stud:
Random: control stud:
Randomised control trial:
Randomized control trial:
Random: control trial:
Randomised crossover stud:
Randomized crossover stud:
Random: crossover stud:

Randomised crossover trial:
Randomized crossover trial:
Random: crossover trial:
Randomised cross-over stud:
Randomized cross-over stud:
Random: cross-over stud:
Randomised cross-over trial:
Randomized cross-over trial:
Random: cross-over trial:
Randomised parallel control stud:
Randomized parallel control stud:
Random: parallel control stud:
Randomised parallel control trial:
Randomized parallel control trial:
Random: parallel control trial:
Randomised parallel controlled stud:
Randomized parallel controlled stud:
Random: parallel controlled stud:
Randomised parallel controlled trial:
Randomized parallel controlled trial:
Random: parallel controlled trial:
Randomised stud:
Randomized stud:
Random: stud:
Randomised trial:
Randomized trial:
Random: trial:
Randomly allocated
Random: allocated
Randomly assigned
Random: assigned
Rate reduction
Relative benefit increas:
Relative benefit reduct:
Relative risk
RR
Relative risk differenc:
Relative risk increas:
Relative risk reduct:
Retrospective stud:
Retrospective trial:
Risk difference:
Risk ratio:
Sham:

Single-blind:
Single mask:
Survival analys:
Therapy trial:
Treatment outcome stud:
Treatment outcome trial:
Treatment stud:
Treatment trial:
Triple-blind:
Triple mask:

Notes on Terms in MEDLINE

Note that with the introduction of publication types in 1990–1991, major changes have occurred in indexing for methodology for therapy studies. Some MeSH terms such as "Randomized controlled trials as topic" (MeSH), have actually changed meanings in the transition to publication types. MeSH indexing and the designation "as topic" in a term indicates articles that are "about" the specific MeSH heading. For example, the MeSH term "Clinical trials as topic" is used when an author writes about the history of clinical trials, describes how to accomplish a certain aspect of clinical trials such as blinding, or is using clinical trials in producing a systematic review article. Publication types describe what something "is"—e.g., an obituary, a bibliography, a review article, a clinical trial, or a randomized controlled trial. Where "dual" terms exist as MeSH and publication types, often the MeSH is in a plural form with the designation "as topic," and the publication type is in the singular form.

Note also that indexers are not consistent with their assignment of MeSH headings and this was shown elegantly in the study by Funk and Reid.[19] Their results can be extrapolated to other databases; therefore, you will likely get better retrieval by combining several index terms and textwords with "ORs" and trying various combinations of the terms, depending on the topic and need. We also encourage you to use the search filters in the next section of the chapter and as described in Chapter 1.

CINAHL (CUMULATIVE INDEX TO NURSING AND ALLIED HEALTH LITERATURE)

Index Terms, Subheadings, and Publication Types

Index Terms

Double-blind studies*
Study design* (can be exploded)

---

*Indicates a preferred term as determined in the Clinical Hedges Study.[20,22]

Treatment outcomes*

"Outcomes (health care)" (can be exploded)
"Process assessment (health care)" (can be exploded)
"Sensitivity and specificity"
Attributable risk
Clinical research (can be exploded)
Clinical trials (can be exploded)
Community trials
Comparative studies
Confidence intervals
Cox proportional hazards model
Crossover design
Epidemiological research (can be exploded)
Evaluation research (can be exploded)
Experimental studies (can be exploded)
Factorial design
Human genome project
Logistic regression (can be exploded)
Medical futility
Meta analysis
Odds ratio
Outcome assessment
Outcomes (can be exploded)
Patient selection
Peer review (can be exploded)
Pilot studies
Placebos
Professional practice, research based (can be exploded)
Prospective studies (can be exploded)
Random assignment
Random sample (can be exploded)
Regression (can be exploded)
Relative risk
Reproducibility of results
Research methodology (can be exploded)
Research (can be exploded)
Retrospective design
Risk assessment
Risk factors (can be exploded)
Sample size
Single-blind studies
Survival analysis (can be exploded)

---

*Indicates a preferred term as determined in the Clinical Hedges Study.[20,22]

Treatment
Treatment failure
Treatment outcomes studies (can be exploded)

Subheadings

Adverse effects
Chemically induced
Contraindications
Diet therapy
Drug therapy
Nursing
Rehamilitation
Radiotherapy
Therapeutic se
Therapy
Surgery

Publication Types

Clinical trial*

Care plan
Case study
Critical path
Diagnostic imagesdrugs
Interview
Nursing diagnoses
Nursing interventions
Practice guidelines
Protocol
Questionnaire
Review
Systematic review

EMBASE

Index Terms, Subheadings, and Publication Types

Index Terms

Clinical trial** (can be exploded)
Health care quality** (can be exploded)

---

*Indicates a preferred term as determined in the Clinical Hedges Study.[23-24]
**Indicates a preferred term as determined in the Clinical Hedges Study.[23]

Treatment outcome* (can be exploded)

Adverse drug reaction (can be exploded)
Cancer survival
Clinical observation
Clinical protocol
Clinical study (can be exploded)
Comparative study (can be exploded)
Crossover procedure
Double blind procedure
Drug efficacy
Evaluation
Experiment (can be exploded)
Factorial analysis
Feasibility study
Follow up
Life expectancy
Longitudinal study
Medical genetics (can be exploded)
Meta analysis
Multicenter study
Observation
Outcomes research
Parallel design
Patient selection
Peer review
Phase 1 clinical trial
Phase 2 clinical trial
Phase 3 clinical trial
Phase 4 clinical trial
Pilot study
Placebo
Prospective study
Randomization
Randomized controlled trial
Regression analysis
Reproducibility
Research (can be exploded)
Retrospective study
Risk (can be exploded)
Risk assessment
Risk factor

---

*Indicates a preferred term as determined in the Clinical Hedges Study.[23]

Sham feeding
Single blind procedure
Statistical model
Survival (can be exploded)
Survival rate
Survival time
Survival
Treatment failure
Types of study (can be exploded)

Subheadings

Adverse drug reaction
Chemically induced
Clinical trial
Disease management
Drug resistance
Drug therapy
Prevention
Radiotherapy
Rehabilitation
Side effect
Surgery
Therapy

Publication Types

None

PsycINFO

Index Terms, Subheadings, and Publication Types

Index Terms

Treatment*

Between groups
Compliance (can be exploded)
Confidence limits, statistics
Dropouts (can be exploded)
Drug tolerance
Effect size, statistical

---

*Indicates a preferred term as determined in the Clinical Hedges Study.[24]

Experiment controls
Experimental attrition
Experimental design (can be exploded)
Experimentation (can be exploded)
Followup studies
Item response theory
Linear regression
Longitudinal studies(can be exploded)
Multiple regression
Nonlinear regression
Placebo
Posttreatment followup
Prevention (can be exploded)
Program evaluation
Prospective studies
Retrospective studies
Risk factors
Sample size
Side effects (can be exploded)
Side effects, drug
Side effects, treatment (can be exploded)
Statistical regression (can be exploded)
Treatment (can be exploded)
Treatment compliance
Treatment dropouts
Treatment duration (can be exploded)
Treatment effectiveness evaluation
Treatment outcomes (can be exploded)

Subheadings

None

Publication Types

Clinical trial
Empirical study
Experimental replication
Followup study
Longitudinal study
Program evaluation
Prospective study
Retrospective study
Treatment outcome study

Notes on Terms in PsycINFO

PsycINFO presents a challenge to those searching for EBHC topics. Unlike MEDLINE, it does not include subheadings which may be attached to descriptors, or free-floated in order to narrow, broaden, or otherwise refine retrieval. Also note that methodology descriptors can indicate that the citation is about the technique or it can indicate the "form" of the research. However, the database does have descriptors which are roughly the conceptual equivalent of MeSH Subheadings. Many of these are broad headings, such as "treatment" (used for therapy), and may be exploded or used in addition to include retrieval from more specific descriptors. *Note:* The explosion function in your vendor's version of PsycINFO may differ in its mechanics from the explosion function in MEDLINE. Consult your database vendor for specifics.

EXAMPLES OF TEXTWORDS AND INDEXING

Example 1

Siedliecki SL, Good M. Effect of music on power, pain, depression and disability. *J Adv Nurs.* 2006;54(5):553–562.

Textwords (in the Title and Abstract of the Article)

Randomized controlled clinical trial
Randomly assigned
Control group

MEDLINE INDEXING

Therapy (floating subheading)
Randomized controlled trial (publication type)

CIHAHL INDEXING

Clinical trials
Random assignment

Example 2

Robinson RG, Jorge RE, Moser DJ, Acion L, Solodkin A, Small SL, Fonzetti P, Hegel M, Arndt S. Escitalopram and problem-solving therapy for prevention of poststroke depression: a randomized controlled trial. *JAMA.* 2008 May 28;299(20):2391–2400.

Textwords (in the Title and Abstract of the Article)

Randomized controlled trial
Placebo
Nonblinded
Intention to treat

MEDLINE INDEXING

Drug therapy subheading
Randomized controlled trial publication type
Multicenter study publication type
Therapeutic use subheading
Prevention and control subheading
Rehabilitation
Double-blind method

CINAHL INDEXING

Therapeutic use subheading
Prevention and control subheading
Rehabilitation subheading
Clinical trial publication type
Research publication type
Methods subheading
Double-blind studies

EMBASE INDEXING

Drug therapy subheading
Prevention subheading
Therapy subheading
Clinical trial
Controlled clinical trial
Controlled study
Double blind procedure
Major clinical study
Multicenter study
Randomized controlled trial
Placebo

PROVEN STRATEGIES

Search Strategies (Filters) Derived during the Clinical Hedges Study[20-24]

Filter*	MEDLINE	CINAHL[†]	EMBASE	PsycINFO
Sensitive	clinical trial.mp. OR clinical trial.pt. OR random:.mp. OR tu (can be exploded)	exp prognosis OR exp study design OR random:.mp.	random:.tw OR clinical trial:.mp. OR exp health care quality	control:.tw. OR random:.tw. OR exp treatment
Specific	randomized controlled trial.pt. OR randomized controlled trial.mp.	double-blind studies.sh. OR random: assignment.mp.	double-blind:.mp. OR placebo:.mp. OR blind:.tw.	double-blind.tw. OR random: assigned:.tw.
Minimize difference between Sensitivity and Specificity	randomized controlled trial.pt. OR randomized.mp. OR placebo.mp.	randomized.tw. OR treatment outcomes.sh. OR clinical trial.pt.	random:.tw. OR placebo:.mp. OR double-blind:.mp.	double-blind.tw. OR random: asigned.tw. OR control.tw.

*See the Introduction for a description of how to use these filters and where to find them in Ovid and PubMed.
[†] In 2009 CINAHL will only be offered through EBSCO. The CINAHL search strategies have been translated and are available for use in EBSCO.

LINKS TO OTHER RESOURCES

Search strategies listing: InterTASC Information Specialists' Sub-Group Search Filter Resource **http://www.york.ac.uk/inst/crd/intertasc/**

EXERCISES

Note that the search possibilities (answers) are detailed in the Appendix.

1. What evidence exists that individualized computer or Internet advice is beneficial to those who wish to lose weight?

2. How strong is the evidence that the establishment of safe injection sites (distribution of needles and provision of a location for people with major substance abuse problems) as described in British Columbia and Australia work at decreasing the spread of diseases?

REFERENCES

1. Moore OA, Smith LA, Campbell F, Seers K, McQuay HJ, Moore RA. Systematic review of the use of honey as a wound dressing. *BMC Complement Altern Med.* 2001;1:2.

2. Jull A, Walker N, Parag V, Molan P, Rogers A, on behalf of the Honey as Adjuvant Leg Ulcer Therapy trial collaborators. Randomized clinical trial of honey-impregnated dressings for venous leg ulcers. *Br J Surg.* 2008;95:175–182.

3. Maizels H, Scott B, Cohen W, Chen W. Intranasal lidocaine for treatment of migraine. A randomized, double-blind, controlled trial. *JAMA.* 1996;276:319–321.

4. Hemila H. Vitamin C, the placebo effects, and the common cold. A case study of how preconceptions influence the analysis of results. *J Clin Epidemiol.* 1996;49:1079–1084.

5. Talbot M. The placebo prescription. *New York Times* Magazine. 2000 January 9. http://www.nytimes.com/library/magazine/home/20000109mag-talbot7.html. Accessed November 24, 2009.

6. Moseley JB, O'Malley K, Petersen, NJ, Menke TJ, Brody BA, Kuykendall D, Hollingsworth HC, Ashton CM, Wray NP. A controlled trial of arthroscopic surgery for osteoarthritis of the knee. *N Engl J Med.* 2002;347:81–88.

7. Christakis GT, Lichtenstein SV, Buth KJ, et al. The influence of risk on the results of warm heart surgery: a substudy of a randomized trial. *Eur J Cardiothorac Surg.* 1997;11:515–520.

8. Chaput de Saintonge DM, Cross KW, Shathorn MK, et al. Hats for the newborn infant. *Br Med J.* 1979;2:570–571.

9. Gwon A. Topical ofloxacin compared with gentamicin in the treatment of external ocular infection. Ofloxacin Study Group. *Br J Ophthalmol.*1992;76:714–718.

10. Frick MH, Elo O, Haapa K, et al. Helinski heart study: primary-prevention trial with gemfibrozil in middle-aged men with dyslipidemia. Safety of treatment, changes in risk factors, and incidence of coronary heart disease. *N Engl J Med.*1987;317:1237–1245.

11. Hux JE, Naylor CD. Communicating the benefits of chronic preventive therapy: does the format of efficacy determine patients acceptance of treatment. *Med Decis Making.*1995;15:152–157.

12. Weintraub DL, Tirumalai EC, Haydel KF, Fujimoto M, Fulton JE, Robinson TN. Team sports for overweight children. The Sanford Sports To Prevent Obesity Randomized Trial. *Arch Ped Adolesc Med.* 2008;162:232–236.

13. Gaede P, Lund-Andersen H, Parving HH, Pedersen O. Effect of a multifactorial intervention on mortality in type 2 diabetes. *N Engl J* Med. 2008;358:580–591.

14. Smith GA, Splaingard M, Hayes JR, Xiang H. Comparison of a personalized parent voice smoke alarm with a conventional residential tone smoke alarm for awaking children. *Pediatrics.* 2006;118:1623–1632.

15. Cohen IT. An overview of the clinical use of ondansetron in preschool age children. *Ther Clin Risk Manag.* 2007;3:333–339.

16. Robinson MH, Hardcastle JD, Moss SM, et al. The risks of screening: Data from the Nottingham randomised controlled trial of faecal occult blood screening for colorectal cancer. *Gut.*1999;45:588–592.

17. Jadad AR. *Randomized Controlled Trials. A User's Guide*. London: *BMJ* Books; 1998.

18. Guyatt G, Rennie D, Mead MO, Cook DJ. *Users' Guides to the Medical Literature. A Manual for Evidence-Based Clinical Practice*, 2nd ed. New York, NY; McGraw-Hill. 2008. Chapter 6. Therapy (Randomized Trials).

19. Funk ME, Reid DA. Indexing consistency in MEDLINE. *Bull Med Libr Assoc.* 1983;71:176–183.

20. Wilczynski NL, Morgan D, Haynes RB; Hedges Team. An overview of the design and methods for retrieving high-quality studies for clinical care. *BMC Med Inform Decis Mak.* 2005;5:20.

21. Haynes RB, McKibbon KA, Wilczynski NL, Walter SD, Werre SR; Hedges Team. Optimal search strategies for retrieving scientifically strong studies of treatment from Medline: analytical survey. *BMJ.* 2005;330(7501):1179.

22. Wong SS, Wilczynski NL, Haynes RB. Optimal CINAHL search strategies for identifying therapy studies and review articles. *J Nurs Scholarsh.* 2006;38:194-199.

23. Wong SS, Wilczynski NL, Haynes RB. Developing optimal search strategies for detecting clinically sound treatment studies in EMBASE. *J Med Libr Assoc.* 2006;94:41-47.

24. Eady AM, Wilczynski NL, Haynes RB. PsycINFO search strategies identified methodologically sound therapy studies and review articles for use by clinicians and researchers. *J Clin Epidemiol.* 2008;61:34-40.

3

Diagnosis and Screening

Nancy Wilczynski

INTRODUCTION

The category of therapy has the most publications of any category of health care research. The second most common type of research is diagnosis. Health professionals are always looking for better ways to determine if diseases or conditions are present in both symptomatic (diagnosis) and asymptomatic (screening) patients. Making an accurate diagnosis is the cornerstone of sound decision making for clinical intervention for health problems—the majority of visits to a family physician are initiated to seek help in understanding a set of signs (signs are those things that we can see; for example, flinching when touching a painful area) and symptoms (symptoms are those things that the patient tells us; for example, the patient is experiencing pain) that might indicate the presence of a disease or disorder. For a diagnostic or screening test to be considered better than what is currently used, the new test would need to give more accurate results, be less risky, less invasive, less expensive, easier to do, less uncomfortable for patients, faster to yield results, technically less challenging, or more easily interpreted.

CLINICAL EXAMPLE

Self-Report Scales in the Diagnosis of Depression in Patients on Hemodialysis

As with the previous chapter, we will start with an example of a problem and the research that went into solving it. The problem was that patients with end-stage renal disease (ESRD) who are treated with hemodialysis may report increased symptoms of fatigue, poor appetite, and sleep disturbance on self-report depression scales that may not be confirmed as a depressive disorder during a structured interview based on the *Diagnostic and Statistical Manual of Mental Disorders IV* (DSM-IV), the gold standard. Self-report depression scales such as the Beck Depression Inventory (BDI) and the Center for Epidemiological Study of Depression (CESD) scale may overemphasize the somatic symptoms of depression and may, therefore, lead to the misclassification of symptoms of uremia and chronic disease for symptoms of depression. A study was needed to explore the diagnostic utility of the BDI and the CESD scale in ESRD patients treated with chronic hemodialysis because, among these patients, depressive symptoms are prevalent and are associated with increased mortality. Hedayati and colleagues[1] undertook such a study and reported their findings in 2006. The aim of the study was to establish the cutoff scores on the BDI and the CESD scale that achieved the best diagnostic accuracy for depression for patients with ESRD.

Ninety-eight consecutive ESRD patients treated with hemodialysis completed the BDI and the CESD scale. A physician blinded to the results of the BDI and CESD scale administered the Structured Clinical Interview for Depression (SCID), a DSM IV-based, well-validated tool for establishing the diagnosis of depressive disorder, the gold standard. Results from the tests (BDI and CESD scale) were compared with results obtained from the gold standard (SCID) on the same patients. Receiver operating characteristic (ROC) curves (defined later in this chapter) were used to determine the best BDI and CESD scale cutoffs for a diagnosis of depression in this patient population. Hedayati and colleagues reported that a cutoff score of 18 and 14 on the CESD scale and the BDI, respectively, achieved the best diagnostic accuracy. That is, for example, patients that had a score above or equal to 18 on the CESD scale were considered to have depression, whereas those with a score below 18 were considered not to have depression. Numerous test characteristics were calculated and presented in the article including that a cutoff of 18 on the CESD scale had a sensitivity of 69%, specificity of 83%, positive predictive value of 60%, negative predictive value of 88%, positive likelihood ratio (+LR) of 4.14, and a negative likelihood ratio (−LR) of 0.37. For the BDI a cutoff score of 14 had a sensitivity of 62%, specificity of 81%, positive predictive value of 53%, negative predictive value of 85%, +LR of 3.26, and −LR of 0.47. All test characteristics are defined later in this chapter using this study in the examples.

The authors of this study concluded that the BDI and the CESD scale did not perform well as diagnostic tools for depression at any cutoff score. However, they additionally concluded that the self-report scales were acceptable screening tools for depression in ESRD patients treated with hemodialysis due to their high +LRs. This knowledge indicates that clinicians who are concerned with the welfare of their patients with ESRD who are on chronic hemodialysis will likely screen for depression periodically using the CESD scale.

HOW DIAGNOSIS STUDIES ARE DONE

The best procedure for evaluating a new diagnostic or screening test involves gathering a group of patients and administering the tests that are to be evaluated. This group should include a **spectrum of patients**, meaning that some but not all patients have the disorder or derangement of interest. Thus, some of the included patients should *not* have the disorder or disease of interest (e.g., depression) while others should have the disease but to differing degrees of severity (e.g., mild, moderate, and severe depression). *Each* person must undergo *both* the currently accepted **gold standard** procedure (often also called the **diagnostic standard** or **criterion standard**) and the new test or tests. Often, the gold standard test is invasive (e.g., surgery or an autopsy to check for the presence of lung cancer), expensive (e.g., a night in a sleep laboratory to evaluate sleep apnea), or time consuming (e.g., a week to culture bronchial lavage fluid to determine whether a patient in the intensive care unit has tuberculosis or pneumonia). The interpretation, or reading, of the gold or diagnostic standard should be done without knowledge of the new test result, *and* the interpretation of the new test should be done without knowledge of the gold or diagnostic standard test result. This is referred to as **blinding** (discussed in the previous chapter).

In this chapter, both diagnosis and screening are covered. Diagnostic tests are used for persons who have signs and symptoms that make the clinician suspicious of the presence of a specific disease or several possible diseases (e.g., cough can indicate a cold, lung cancer, whooping cough, or an adverse reaction to some antihypertension medications). Screening tests are done for persons who have no clinical signs or symptoms for the disease being tested (e.g., mammographies to detect breast cancer in all women over the age of 50 years). Both diagnostic and screening tests are evaluated using the same testing methodology, and the results are presented using the same terminology and statistics. "Good" tests are ones that give positive results when the disease or condition is present *and* give negative results when the disease or condition is absent. Measures of the "positive-when-should-be-positive" and "negative-when-should-be-negative" are called the **test characteristics**, and are described below. Briefly, the characteristics are sensitivity and specificity; positive and negative likelihood ratios; positive and negative predictive values; and false positive and false negative rates.

2 X 2 TABLE

Often, data from the evaluation of a screening or diagnostic test are presented in a **2 × 2 table** (or **2 by 2 table**). The **"truth"** or **gold standard results** go across the top of the table, and the new test results go down the left-hand side of the table. Pictorially it has the structure shown in Table 3-1, with the boxes, or **data cells,** labeled *a, b, c,* and *d.* For example, in the 2 × 2 table shown in Table 3-1, the number of persons listed in box or cell *a* is the number of persons who have a positive result using the gold standard test *and* a positive result using the new test being evaluated. **Cell *a*** can also be called the **number of true positives**—the test is positive and correct in that the patient has the disease. **Cell *d*** is the **number of true negatives**, a negative result when using the gold standard test *and* a negative result when using the new test being evaluated—the test is negative and correct in that the patient does not have the disease. **Cell *b*** is the **number of false positives**, a negative result using the gold standard test *and* a positive result using the new test being evaluated—you do not have the disease but are told that you do. **Cell *c*** is the **number of false negatives**, a positive result using the gold standard test *and* a negative result using the new test being evaluated—the patient has the disease but is told that he/she does not. Data in the four cells *a* through *d* are used to calculate the test characteristics shown in Table 3-1.

Table 3-1.

| | Disease/Condition (Gold Standard) | | |
| | Positive | Negative | |
	+	–	
New test + Positive results	a	b	a + b
New test – Negative results	c	d	c + d
	a + c	b + d	a + b + c + d

Sensitivity = a/(a + c)
Specificity = d/(b + d)
Positive predictive value = a/(a + b)
Negative predictive value = d/(c + d)
Positive likelihood ratio = sensitivity/(100 − specificity)
Negative likelihood ratio = (100 − sensitivity)/specificity
False positive rate = 100 − specificity *or* b/(b + d)
False negative rate = 100 − sensitivity *or* c/(a + c)

DEFINITIONS

The testing of diagnostic procedures initially looks fairly straightforward. It is, however, the clinical research methodology that has the most jargon. Researchers compare the results of the old (or gold standard) test (positive and negative) with the results of the new test (positive and negative). They do this to ensure that the new test results are correct as often as possible; that is, the new test results are positive when they should be positive *and* negative when they should be negative.

Sensitivity and Specificity

The two most frequently used measures of this correctness are the sensitivity and specificity of the test. **Sensitivity** measures the proportion of patients with the disease or disorder of interest as defined by the gold standard who have a positive test result. One example of a test that has high sensitivity is the standard pregnancy test based on biochemical analysis of hormone levels (Table 3-2). The test correctly detects a very large proportion of the patients who are pregnant. Using the data from Table 3-2, the new test has a sensitivity of 92%, calculated using the formula $a/(a + c)$ or 23/25. In our clinical example summarized at the beginning of this chapter, the CESD scale had a sensitivity of 69% for detecting depression in ESRD patients when using a cutoff score of 18. This means that 69% of the patients with depression as defined by the gold standard were considered to have depression based on the results of the new test, the CESD scale, a low figure when you are considering the CESD scale as a new diagnostic tool.

Table 3-2.
Example Using Data Comparing Pregnancy Tests of 100 Women

| | Pregnancy (test repeated over time) | | | | |
	Positive +	Negative −			
New test + Positive results	23 a	b 0	a + b		23
New test − Negative results	2 c	d 75	c + d		77
	25 a + c	b + d 75	a + b + c + d		100

The **specificity** of the test measures the proportion of patients without the disorder or condition of interest as defined by the gold standard who have a negative test result. The standard biochemical pregnancy test has a very high specificity. The specificity is 100%, calculated using the formula $d/(b + d)$ or 75/75 (see Table 3-2). When the specificity is extremely high, a positive test result will rule in the disease or condition; in other words, in this case, if the test is positive the woman is pregnant. In our clinical example, the CESD scale had a specificity of 83% when using a cutoff score of 18. This means that 83% of the patients without depression as defined by the gold standard test were not considered to have depression based on the results of the new test, the CESD scale.

Both sensitivity and specificity must be high for a diagnostic test to be truly useful in a clinical setting. In practice, both sensitivity and specificity should be over 80% for a clinically useful test. For screening tests, such as the prostate-specific antigen test to detect prostate cancer in asymptomatic men, specificity should be close to perfect (100%) to avoid incorrectly telling people without the disorder that they do indeed have cancer. Currently, no test has a sensitivity *and* a specificity of 100%. Often, if the test result level is adjusted to maximize the sensitivity, the specificity will fall, and if the test result level is changed to maximize the specificity, the sensitivity will fall.

Positive Predictive Value and Negative Predictive Value

Other measures of the "worth" or performance of a diagnostic or screening test are the positive and the negative predictive values. These are measures of what either a positive or negative test result actually tells us about the probability of the disease or disorder in question for the specific setting in which the test was evaluated. **Positive predictive value** is the proportion of patients with a positive test result who have the disease or condition in question. **Negative predictive value** is the proportion of patients with a negative test result who do not have the disease or condition in question. The positive predictive value of the new pregnancy test for the 100 women in our sample shown in Table 3-2 is very high at 100%, calculated using the formula a/(a + b) or 23/23. This means that; if the test result is positive, a woman almost certainly is pregnant. The test has a smaller negative predictive value at 97%, calculated using the formula d/(d + c) or 75/77. A test may be negative because a woman is truly not pregnant, or simply because her reproductive system has not had enough time to produce sufficient hormone levels to test positive. In our clinical example the positive and negative predictive values for the CESD scale at a cutoff score of 18 were 60% and 88%, respectively. This means that 60% of the patients considered to have depression based on the results of the new test, the CESD scale, had depression as defined by the gold standard, and 88% of the patients considered not to have depression based on the results of the new test did not have depression as defined by the gold standard.

Predictive values are affected by the **prevalence** of the target disorder in the population being studied. For diagnostic/screening test evaluation, prevalence is the proportion of patients with the target disorder or the disease in question among all tested patients. Prevalence is also sometimes called **pretest probability** or **pretest likelihood** of the target disorder, disease, or condition. Considering two populations of patients with different pretest likelihoods for pulmonary embolism illustrates the effect that prevalence can have on predictive values. One population includes elderly patients who developed pleuritic chest pain after a complete hip replacement and who had not been given prophylactic anticoagulants to prevent blood clots. These blood clots can lead to pulmonary embolism or deep venous thrombosis, which can be fatal. The second population includes young men with similar chest pain that developed while they were playing baseball. Although the tests both groups would receive have identical sensitivity and specificity values, the positive and negative predictive values would be different, because the pretest likelihood (prevalence) of pulmonary embolism would be much higher in elderly patients after surgery than in young men after baseball.

Likelihood Ratios

Likelihood ratios, both positive and negative (**+LR and −LR**), are other measures of a test's worth or performance. LRs incorporate both the sensitivity and specificity of the test and indicate how much the probability of disease changes from baseline (i.e., before the test) when the test result is positive (+LR) or negative (−LR). +LRs tell you how much the odds of the disease increase when a test is positive. Useful tests will have larger +LRs and less useful tests will have smaller +LRs. The further the LR is from 1, the more it changes the probability of disease. +LRs are taken seriously when they are in the range of 2 or more, and are clinically useful when they are greater than 5. A test with a +LR of 24 means that a positive test result is 24 times more likely to have come from a person with the disorder of interest than from a person without the disorder. −LRs tell you how much the odds of the disease decrease when a test is negative. Useful tests will have −LRs close to 0, and less useful tests will have higher −LRs. For −LRs the numbers that deserve attention are less than 0.1. For a more thorough summary of making sense of diagnostic test results using LRs see the article by Richardson and colleagues.[2] Another way to look at LRs is the higher the +LR, the more likely the patient will have a positive test result if he/she has the disorder; the lower the −LR, the less likely the patient will have a positive test result if he/she does not have the disorder.

The new pregnancy test we are considering has a +LR of infinity, calculated as sensitivity/(100 − specificity) or 92/(100 − 100) (see Table 3-2); therefore, any woman who has a positive test is infinitely more likely to be pregnant than if she had received a negative test result. The −LR of 0.08, calculated as (100 − sensitivity)/specificity or 100 − 92/100 (see Table 3-2), means that a woman with a negative test has 4 chances in 50 (or 8 in 100) of being pregnant (or 46 chances out of 50 of not being pregnant). In our clinical example, the +LR was 4.14 for the CESD scale at a cutoff score of 18. This means that a positive test result (i.e., scoring 18 or higher on the CESD scale) is just over 4 times more likely to have come from a patient with depression as defined by the gold standard than from a patient without depression. The −LR was 0.37, which means that a patient with a negative test result (i.e., scoring less than 18 on the CESD scale) has about a 1 chance in 3 (or 37 in 100) of having depression, not an encouraging result for a diagnostic test. Based on these

LRs, the authors of the study concluded that the CESD scale was not a good diagnostic tool (high −LR) but would be acceptable as a screening tool for depression at the proposed cutoff score of 18 (high +LR).

The "beauty" of LRs is that they take information from the patient in question and the clinical situation and use the information to understand that person's individual probably of disease depending on the test results. LRs are combined with information about the prevalence of the disease, characteristics of a patient pool, and information about a particular patient to determine the post-test odds of the disease. For instance, in interpreting the test results for a specific patient, a clinician must take into account how likely he/she thinks the patient sent for testing is to have the disease or condition before testing and then apply this pretest likelihood to the final test results (i.e., the pretest likelihood is multiplied by the +LR or −LR depending on whether the test result for the patient is positive or negative giving the post-test odds of having the disease). A fuller explanation of the usefulness of likelihood ratios is contained in an editorial by Sackett and Straus.[3] Described in another fashion, LRs "start" with the patient's probability of disease (a given number) and then, using the test results (positive or negative), the clinician can then calculate how likely that person is to have the disease based on these results—decisions can then be made to stop the diagnostic process (low probability of disease), initiate treatment (high probability of disease), or continue doing testing (intermediate probability of disease).

False Positive Rate and False Negative Rate

Two other test definitions less often used are false positive rate and false negative rate. For the pregnancy test the **false positive rate** is 0%, calculated as 100 − specificity or 100 − 100 (see Table 3-2). This is the proportion of women who received a positive test result when they were truly not pregnant. The **false negative rate** is the proportion of women who received a negative test result when they are truly pregnant. For the pregnancy test, the false negative rate is 8%, calculated as 100 − sensitivity or 100 − 92 = 8 (see Table 3-2). False positive and false negative test results both affect people's lives. With a false positive test result, people assume incorrectly that they have the disease or condition for which they were tested and become "labeled." People who think they are sick can actually start acting unwell even though they are healthy. They may miss time from work or refuse promotions and their general quality of life may deteriorate. A study by Johnston et al[4] showed that this happened to men working in a steel mill after being told incorrectly that they had high blood pressure. False negative test results also affect people's lives. People who are given false negative test results may not seek treatment when they should. For example, valuable treatment time is lost if the woman with breast cancer is told she does not have a malignancy when she really does.

One other way to describe this set of numbers is the number of false positive and the number of false negative patients in the group. The number of false positives is the number in the cell *b* of the 2 × 2 table and the number of false negatives is the number in cell *c* of the 2 × 2 table; in our example these are 0 and 2, respectively (see Table 3-2).

RECEIVER OPERATING CHARACTERISTIC CURVES

Receiver operating (or operator) characteristic (ROC) curves are graphic representations of diagnostic test comparisons when the test results can have ranges of values (e.g., different cutoff scores on the CESD scale). Using cardiac enzyme levels to diagnose myocardial infarction or various values for fasting blood glucose levels in persons who are suspected of having diabetes mellitus are examples where ROC curves can be useful. If the test has more than one possible cut point (laboratory value, test score), or has a range of two or more test values, (for example, negative, weakly positive, and strongly positive), a ROC curve can be made by plotting sensitivity (the true positive rate on the *y*-axis) and 1 − specificity (the false positive rate on the *x*-axis) on a graph. Each point on the graph, then, has its own sensitivity and specificity value. A "good" test will have a ROC value (area under the curve) of >80%; that is, a curve that "climbs" steeply and approaches the top quickly before it levels off. Calculations are often done to find out what point or position on the curve (laboratory value, test score) has the best combination of sensitivity and specificity.

Clinicians who make health care decisions should learn how to interpret the above mentioned test characteristics. For others, especially librarians who use the terms for building search strategies to aid in information retrieval, it is not as essential to learn the precise definitions of the terms. Most standard texts have definitions. Most articles evaluating diagnostic tests report the sensitivity and specificity of the tests. LRs are being reported more frequently now than in the past and have several advantages over sensitivity and specificity; for example, they are less likely to change with the prevalence of the disorder, they can be calculated for several levels of cut points of the test, they can be used to combine the results of multiple diagnostic tests, and they can be used to calculate the post-test probability of a target disorder or condition.

UNDERSTANDING DIAGNOSTIC STATISTICS

Most clinicians do not routinely calculate their own test characteristics for diagnostic tests, but completing a set of calculations may make understanding the concepts easier. We will proceed using a clinical scenario of a 35-year-old woman who may have acute pancreatitis. Our diagnostic

Table 3-3.
2 X 2 Table for the Diagnosis of Pancreatitis: Worksheet

Disease/condition: _____
Gold standard: _____

	Positive +	Negative −	
New test+ Positive results	a	b	a + b
New test − Negative results	c	d	c + d
	a + c	b + d	a + b + c + d

Sensitivity = a/(a + c)
= ___/(___ + ___)
= ___/___
= _____

Specificity = d/(b + d)
= ___/(___ + ___)
= ___/___
= _____

Positive likelihood ratio = sensitivity/(100 − specificity)
= _____/(100 − _____)
= _____/_____
= _____

Negative likelihood ratio = (100 − sensitivity)/specificity
= (100 − _____/(_____)
= _____/_____
= _____

Positive predictive value = a/(a + b)
= ___/(___ + ___)
= ___/___
= _____

Negative predictive value = d/(c + d)
= ___/(___ + ___)
= ___/___
= _____

False positive rate = 100 − specificity
= 100 − (___)
= _____

False negative rate = 100 − specificity
= 100 − (___)
= _____

suspicion is high. Her symptoms include epigastric pain, anorexia, vomiting, nausea, and fever, and she has a history of alcohol abuse. Using data from a book of diagnostic strategies by Panzer and colleagues[5] to study a population of 200 persons with suspected pancreatitis, all would be given a new test, a serum lipase test. To evaluate whether the serum lipase test is a valid test (sensitivity and specificity over 80%), the results of the lipase test were compared with the diagnostic standard. An effective diagnostic standard for many diseases, including this one, is careful observation of the patient over time to determine whether the disease develops. The charts of all 200 persons were checked within 3 months, and each person was contacted by telephone to see if he/she had had pancreatitis. Both the chart reviewers and the telephone interviewers did not know the results of the lipase test for a given patient (blinding). For the 200 persons tested, the chart audit and telephone contact showed that 53 had had pancreatitis and 147 did not. Of the 53 people with pancreatitis, the lipase test was positive for 50 of the participants; 7 patients without pancreatitis had a positive lipase test. Fill in the worksheet on p. 64 (Table 3-3) and calculate the sensitivity and specificity, positive and negative LRs, positive and negative predictive values, and false positive and negative rates for the serum lipase test. The answers follow.

Table 3-4.
2 X 2 Table for the Diagnosis of Pancreatitis: Answers

	Disease/condition: Pancreatitis (gold standard): Watchful waiting				
	Positive +		Negative −		
New test: **serum lipase test** + Positive results	50 a	b	7	a + b	57
New test: **serum lipase test** − Negative results	3 c	d	140	c + d	143
	53 a + c	b + d	147	a + b + c + d	200

Sensitivity = a/(a + c)
 = 50/(50 + 3)
 = 50/53
 = 94% or 0.94

Specificity = d/(b + d)
 = 140/(7 + 140)
 = 140/147
 = 95% or 0.95

Positive LR = sensitivity/(100 − specificity)
 = 94/(100 − 95)
 = 94/5
 = 18.8

Negative LR = (100 − sensitivity)/specificity
 = (100 − 94)/95
 = 6/95
 = 0.06

Positive Predictive Value = a/(a + b)
 = 50/(50 + 7)
 = 50/57
 = 88%

Negative Predictive Value = d/(c + d)
 = 140/(3 + 140)
 = 140/143
 = 98%

False Positive Rate = 100 − specificity
 = 100 − 95
 = 5%

False Negative Rate = 100 − sensitivity
 = 100 − 94
 = 6%

SUMMARY

In summary, diagnostic and screening test evaluations are done using a methodology that incorporates the following features (in the order of importance, from most to least important) that the Evidence-Based Medicine Working Group has designated in their User's Guide series[6]:

- The laboratory or research personnel who administer and evaluate or read the tests should be blinded to the results of the other tests being compared.
- The patient group should include persons with a spectrum of disease, from no disease to severe disease (often a large group of persons, not all of whom may have had the disease).
- A diagnostic or gold standard test already exists (e.g., biopsy or a night in a sleep laboratory).
- Every person involved in the evaluation receives all the tests that are being evaluated. The order in which they receive the tests can be in random order, fixed order, or by convenience of the testing personnel or patients. Sets of test results for the new and old tests are compared for being positive when the test results should be positive *and* negative when the test results should be negative.
- These agreements (i.e., positive with positive and negative with negative) are measured using paired terms of sensitivity and specificity, positive and negative likelihood ratios, positive and negative predictive values, and false and negative test rates.

SEARCHING METHODOLOGY

Now that we have summarized the components of diagnostic test evaluation we move onto searching for diagnostic studies in the large electronic databases such as MEDLINE. This task can be challenging but using search terms that target the methodology specific to diagnostic and screening test evaluations in addition to content terms (e.g., depression) can aid in retrieval effectiveness. The search terms available in 4 of the large electronic databases follow. The terms were compiled during the Clinical Hedges Study[7] after seeking input from clinicians and librarians in the United States and Canada. Index terms, subheadings, and publication types are assigned to each article in the database by staff working for the electronic database (e.g., MEDLINE). Textwords are used to search for articles using the article title and the article abstract. Preferred search terms are shown for MEDLINE and EMBASE as search strategies were developed for detecting diagnostic studies during the Clinical Hedges Study for these 2 databases.

MEDLINE

MeSH, Subheadings, Publication Types, and Textwords

MeSH (Medical Subject Headings — Index Terms)

Diagnosis* (can be exploded)
Diagnosis, differential*
Diagnostic techniques and procedures (can be exploded)*
Predictive value of tests*
Sensitivity and specificity (can be exploded)*

Area under curve
Bayes theorem
Diagnosis, computer assisted (can be exploded)
Diagnosis, dual (psychiatry)
Diagnostic errors (can be exploded)
False negative reactions
False positive reactions
Genetic testing
Laboratory techniques and procedures (can be exploded)
Likelihood functions
Mandatory testing
Mass chest x-ray
Mass screening (can be exploded)
Multiphasic screening
Neonatal screening
Observer variation
Odds ratio
Probability (can be exploded)
Reference standards
ROC curve
Substance abuse detection
Vision screening

Subheadings

Diagnosis* (for diagnosis of diseases and disorders) (can be exploded)*

Diagnostic use (for substances used in diagnosis)

Publication Types

None

---

*Indicates a preferred term as determined in the Clinical Hedges Study.[8]

Textwords (Same List Is Used for All 4 Databases)

Accurac:* (combination of sensitivity and specificity)
Accuracy*
Diagnos:*
Predictive value:*
Sensitiv:*
Specificit:*

Area under the curve:
Criterion standard:
Diagnostic standard:
False negative
False positive
False rate:
Gold standard:
Likelihood ratio:
Post test likelihood
Posttest likelihood
Post test probability
Posttest probability
Pre test likelihood
Pretest likelihood
Receiver operat: curve:
ROC

CINAHL (CUMULATIVE INDEX TO NURSING AND ALLIED HEALTH LITERATURE)

Index Terms, Subheadings, and Publication Types

Index Terms

Clinical assessment tools (can be exploded)
Comparative studies
Diagnosis (can be exploded)
Diagnosis, cardiovascular (can be exploded)
Diagnosis, computer assisted (can be exploded)
Diagnosis, delayed
Diagnosis, developmental (can be exploded)
Diagnosis, differential
Diagnosis, digestive system (can be exploded)
Diagnosis, dual (psychiatry)

---

*Indicates a preferred term as determined in the Clinical Hedges Study.[8,9]

Diagnosis, endocrine (can be exploded)
Diagnosis, eye (can be exploded)
Diagnosis, laboratory (can be exploded)
Diagnosis, musculoskeletal (can be exploded)
Diagnosis, neurologic (can be exploded)
Diagnosis, ob-gyn (can be exploded)
Diagnosis, oral (can be exploded)
Diagnosis, otorhinolaryngologic (can be exploded)
Diagnosis, psychosocial (can be exploded)
Diagnosis, radioisotope (can be exploded)
Diagnosis, respiratory system (can be exploded)
Diagnosis, surgical (can be exploded)
Diagnosis, urologic (can be exploded)
Diagnostic errors (can be exploded)
Diagnostic imaging (can be exploded)
Diagnostic reasoning
Diagnostic tests, routine
False negative results
False positive results
Genetic screening
Health screening (can be exploded)
Mandatory testing
Maximum likelihood
Measurement issues and assessments (can be exploded)
Nursing assessment
Nursing diagnosis
Observer bias (can be exploded)
Odds ratio
Precision
Predictive value of tests
Probability
Reproducibility of results
Sensitivity and specificity
Substance abuse detection (can be exploded)
Validity (can be exploded)
Vision screening

Subheadings

Diagnosis
Radiography
Ultrasonography
Diagnostic use
Nursing
Symptoms

Publication Types

Diagnostic images

EMBASE

Index Terms, Subheadings, and Publication Types

Index Terms

Diagnosis* (can be exploded)
Diagnostic accuracy*
Diagnostic error*
Diagnostic procedure* (can be exploded)
Diagnostic test* (can be exploded)
Diagnostic value*

Accuracy
Area under the curve
Bayes theorem
Classification (can be exploded)
Coding and classification (can be exploded)
Computer assisted diagnosis (can be exploded)
Differential diagnosis
Discriminant analysis
Disease classification (can be exploded)
Genetic screening
Laboratory diagnosis (can be exploded)
Mass screening (can be exploded)
Maximum likelihood method
Newborn screening
Nomogram
Observer variation
Pharmacokinetics (can be exploded)
Probability
Psychiatric diagnosis (can be exploded)
Receiver operating characteristic
Screening test
Sensitivity and specificity
Screening (can be exploded)
Substance abuse
Thorax radiography
Vision test (can be exploded)

*Indicates a preferred term as determined in the Clinical Hedges Study.[9]

Visual system examination (can be exploded)

Subheadings

Diagnosis*

Diagnostic use

Publication Types

None

PsycINFO

Index Terms, Subheadings, and Publication Types

Index Terms

Computer assisted diagnosis (can be exploded)
Criterion referenced test
Diagnosis (can be exploded)
Differential diagnosis
Dual diagnosis
Health screening (can be exploded)
Medical diagnosis (can be exploded)
Misdiagnosis
Neuropsychological assessment (can be exploded)
Prenatal diagnosis
Probability (can be exploded)
Psychodiagnosis (can be exploded)
Psychodiagnostic interview (can be exploded)
Psychodiagnostic typologies (can be exploded)
Psychological screening inventory
Screening tests (can be exploded)
Screening (can be exploded)
Statistical probability (can be exploded)
Symptom checklists
Taxonomies

Subheadings

None

Publication Types

None

*Indicates a preferred term as determined in the Clinical Hedges Study.[9]

EXAMPLES OF TEXTWORDS AND INDEXING USING OUR CLINICAL EXAMPLE

Citation for Our Clinical Example

Hedayati SS, Bosworth HB, Kuchibhatla M, Kimmel PL, Szczech LA. The predictive value of self-report scales compared with physician diagnosis of depression in hemodialysis patients. Kidney Int 2006;69:1662-1668.

Textwords and Index Terms Used in Our Clinical Example

Textwords (in the Title and Abstract of the Article)

Accurac:*
Accuracy*
Diagnos:*
Predictive value:*
Sensitiv:*
Specificity*

Likelihood ratio:
Receiver operat: curve:
Specificit:

MEDLINE INDEXING

Diagnosis* (subheading)

CINAHL INDEXING

Diagnosis (subheading)

EMBASE INDEXING

Diagnosis* (subheading)
Diagnostic accuracy*
Diagnostic value*

Receiver operating characteristic
Sensitivity and specificity

---

*Indicates a preferred term as determined in the Clinical Hedges Study.[8,9]

PROVEN STRATEGIES

Search Strategies (Filters) Derived during the Clinical Hedges Study[8,9]

Filter*	MEDLINE (Ovid syntax)	EMBASE (Ovid syntax)
Sensitive	sensitiv:.mp. OR diagnos:.mp. OR di.fs.	di.fs. OR predict:.tw. OR specificity.tw.
Specific	specificity.tw.	specificity.tw.
Minimize difference between Sensitivity and Specificity	sensitiv:.mp. OR predictive value:.mp. OR accurac:.tw.	sensitiv:.tw. OR diagnostic accuracy.sh. OR diagnostic.tw.

*See the Introduction for a description of how to use these filters and where to find them in Ovid and PubMed.

LINKS TO OTHER RESOURCES

Link to information regarding the Clinical Hedges Study:
http://hiru.mcmaster.ca/hiru/HIRU_Hedges_home.aspx

Link to how to use an article about a diagnostic test:
http://www.cche.net/usersguides/diagnosis.asp

EXERCISES

Note that the search possibilities (answers) are detailed in the Appendix.

1. Can short questionnaires be used to detect anxiety disorders in primary care?
2. Can plasma fatty acid analysis be used in the diagnosis of cystic fibrosis?

REFERENCES

1. Hedayati SS, Bosworth HB, Kuchibhatla M, Kimmel PL, Szczech LA. The predictive value of self-report scales compared with physician diagnosis of depression in hemodialysis patients. *Kidney Int.* 2006;69:1662-1668.
2. Richardson WS, Wilson MC, Keitz SA, Wyer PC; EBM Teaching Scripts Working Group. Tips for teachers of evidence-based medicine: Making sense of diagnostic test results using likelihood ratios. *J Gen Intern Med.* 2006;23:87-92.
3. Sackett DL, Straus S. On some clinically useful measures of the accuracy of diagnostic testing. *ACP J Club.* 1998;129:A17-19.

4. Johnston ME, Gibson ES, Terry CW, et al. Effects of labelling on income, work and social function among hypertensive employees. *J Chronic Dis*. 1984;37:417-423.

5. Panzer RJ, Black ER, Griner PF, eds. *Diagnostic Strategies for Common Medical Problems*. Philadelphia, PA: American College of Physicians; 1991:160.

6. Guyatt G, Rennie D, Meade MO, Cook DJ. *Users' Guide to the Medical Literature. A Manual for Evidence-Based Clinical Practice*. 2nd ed. New York, NY: McGraw-Hill Co; 2008 (chapter on diagnosis).

7. Wilczynski NL, Morgan D, Haynes RB; Hedges Team. An overview of the design and methods for retrieving high-quality studies for clinical care. *BMC Med Inform Decis Mak*. 2005;5:20.

8. Haynes RB, Wilczynski NL. Optimal search strategies for retrieving scientifically strong studies of diagnosis from Medline: analytical survey. *BMJ*. 2004;328:1040.

9. Wilczynski NL, Haynes RB; Hedges Team. EMBASE search strategies for identifying methodologically sound diagnostic studies for use by clinicians and researchers. *BMC Med*. 2005;3:7.

4

Etiology, Causation, and Harm

Ann McKibbon

INTRODUCTION

Another very important area of health care research is **etiology** or **causation**—questions regarding "why" or "how did this happen?" An alternative term for this area of health research is **harm**. This area is concerned with assessing whether a condition or situation such as asbestos or drinking water high in aluminum content are contributing factors to the development of lung cancer or Alzheimer disease, respectively. The terms *etiology* and *causation* are associated with the development of conditions or diseases, while the term *harm* is often used when clinicians refer to drug and other interventional studies and the adverse effects that can develop. Assessment of etiology, causation, or harm is becoming more important as people become aware of the choices they have in relation to prevention and control of diseases and conditions. As in the therapy chapter (Chapter 2), one can study the issues of "causing" both good and bad things to happen. Often, the topics of etiology and causation are long-term issues, such as maternal well being during pregnancy affecting the well being of the fetus and the mental health of the child as it grows; exercise during adulthood decreasing the risk for osteoporosis in women after menopause; or if exposure to electromagnetic energy fields from electric power lines causes leukemia in children.

FOUR METHODOLOGIES FOR EVALUATING ETIOLOGY

Briefly, 2 components are included and evaluated in causation studies: assessments of exposures or risk factors and the related disease or condition outcomes. For example, does having dental fillings that contain mercury, owning pets early in life, living in cooler climates, having had optic neuritis, or being a young woman (the risk factors or exposures) increase one's risk for developing multiple sclerosis (the outcomes)? At various times, researchers have felt that all of these factors might be related to an increased risk for multiple sclerosis. Conversely, the following factors have been considered to be "protective" or to reduce the risk for development of multiple sclerosis: no pets during childhood, no dental caries, living in tropical climates, not having had optic neuritis, or being a man. For the purposes of this book we will assume that etiology refers to both the increased risk for development and protection against a disease or condition.

Not everyone, however, agrees with both the increased risk and protective factors being called "causation." Indexers who produce MEDLINE and other databases often separate the two issues of increased risk and protective factors into distinct categories: Indexers for MEDLINE consider the study of increased risk to be "etiology" and the protective effects to be "prevention and control." This has implications for building search strategies to address clinical questions of etiology.

People working with etiology/causation questions often describe their work with exposures and outcomes as seeking to determine if "associations" exist between the 2. An association is considered to be present if 2 or more things happen or occur at the same time. The association can be positive— both things together are increasing or decreasing; e.g., more smoking accelerates the rate of development of lung cancer. The association can also be negative, an example of which would be the more one exercises, the less one's chance for developing cardiovascular disorders. A strong association is the first step toward determining if the exposure does cause the outcome rather than just both occurring at the same time.

Well-done etiology studies that provide strong evidence of causation are commonly complex and consume substantial time and resources. Often ethical and resource issues dictate that a variety of methods across a series of studies are needed to fully address and understand many causation topics. Etiology research can be done using at least 4 different methodologies. Their strength of evidence, time point when the exposures and outcomes are assessed, and relative frequency of publication are shown pictorially in Table 4-1. The 4 methods vary in many aspects, most importantly in their strength of evidence and frequency of publication. Generally, studies with the highest methodological quality or strength of evidence are clustered at the narrowest part of the publishing wedge: they are the most appropriate for use in clinical decision making.

Because multiple approaches are needed to assess cause and effect, etiology is probably one of the most complex, if not the most difficult, of the clinical categories to understand and apply. The best way to begin to understand and compare the 4 methods is to start with a concrete clinical example and work with it while referring to the features listed in Table 4-1.

Table 4-1.
Study Designs Used in Etiology Research Showing Methods Used, Strength of Evidence, Time of Exposure, and Frequency of Publication

Methodology	Strength of Evidence	Time of Exposure	Frequency of Publication
Randomized controlled trials	Strong	Future	Very few
Cohort studies	Moderate	Present	Some
Case-control studies	Useful but weaker	Past	Moderate number
Cross-sectional studies with statistically adjusted groups	Weakest	Variable and often cannot tell because both exposure and outcomes are assessed at the same point in time	Very many in relation to the other types of etiology studies

CLINICAL EXAMPLE

Does Your Spouse's Occupation, Job Status, and Salary Affect Your Mortality, and Do These Same Features for You Affect Your Spouse's Mortality?

Anecdotally, certainly in my circle of friends and relatives, people feel that their spouse can affect their health and well being. How can the evidence on this topic be studied?

For simplicity's sake we will choose to study 3 "exposures": the spouse's education, job status, and income. As an "outcome," we will evaluate only mortality. Mortality is an outcome that is relatively easy to ascertain. Mortality is also relatively easy to define (as compared to happiness, job satisfaction, family rearing success, and similar quality-of-life measures). Mortality is well tracked by all countries and their jurisdictions (e.g., states, provinces, municipalities, and regions) and reporting is standardized world-wide. We will start with the top of the table (randomized controlled trials) and move downward, covering cohort, case-control, and cross-sectional studies considering if the study methods are reasonable and do-able.

Randomized Controlled Trials

Using the strongest methodology, the **randomized controlled trial**, we would have to assemble a group of men and women (or couples) and randomly allocate them to various educational levels, occupations, and incomes. Alternatively we could randomly allocate people to marriage partners. This project would involve a long period of time, many sub-studies or a study that was very complex that could evaluate the effect of these 3 factors (educational level, job status, and income) on our outcome of choice—mortality. We would have to wait a long period of time to determine the effect of education, job, and income on mortality. Common sense tells us that a randomized controlled trial method would be almost impossible to do, cost an absolutely huge amount of money, interfere far too much in peoples' lives, and take almost 50 years to complete. We need to move on to other methods to reliably and realistically answer our question of spousal socioeconomic factors affecting our mortality.

Cohort Studies

The next strongest methodology for testing etiology questions is the **cohort study**. The term *cohort* comes from the Latin word for "group": a cohort was a unit of a Roman army, equivalent to several hundred men. Cohort studies follow a group of people over time and measure outcomes. Researchers gather people who do not have the outcome of interest, such as recurrent otitis media in preschool children. They then ascertain which children in the cohort or group have been or are being exposed to the possible causative agent: in this case, secondhand tobacco-smoke exposure (having parents and other adult members of the households who smoke). After a period of time of following how the children in the cohort groups are faring, the research staff compares the number of children in each group (the group with exposure to secondhand smoke and the group without exposure) that have developed the disease in question (ear infections). Evidence does support that children who are exposed to secondhand smoke do have a higher rate of otitis media. A cohort study can start "now" collecting data on exposures and outcomes or it can use data from the past.

A cohort study of the question of spousal education, occupation, and income would start by collecting data on these 3 risk factors in married men and women and follow them forward in time to collect data on mortality and at what age it occurred. Because the time between exposure to one's spouse and his or her socioeconomic situation and mortality is often a long one, this study would take considerable time unless data had been collected retrospectively (back in time).

Because we do not "control" who has the exposures, cohort studies are more difficult to analyze appropriately and researchers are more careful in reporting and applying their results. In cohort studies one must look for and factor in bias and confounders. **Bias** is defined as any factor that can take us away from the truth either consciously or unconsciously. Biases can be systematic (taking us away from the truth in one direction) or random (taking us away from the truth in multiple unknowable directions). **Confounders** are complex factors or occurrences that affect both the outcome and the exposures. An example of a common confounder is alcohol drinking in smoking studies. Smoking can also be a confounder in alcohol studies. People who smoke often drink and people who drink also often smoke. To illustrate these 2 confounders a study might ascertain that smoking is linked to divorces—the rate of divorce is higher in smokers. Further analyses of the drinking habits of participants may determine that drinking is linked to both smoking and to divorce. This confounding by the drinking clouds the true picture of the interaction between smoking and divorce.

Both bias and confounders must be determined as carefully and accurately as possible and then used in the data collection and final analyses. In our study a confounder may be something like pre-existing disease such as diabetes, severe asthma, or congenital heart defects that might affect both the choice of profession and salary (lower because the person cannot work), as well as choice of partner and mortality. Biases are simpler to understand and often more common. For example, detection bias occurs when we think we should be finding "something" and we continue to look for it even if it is not there. If one continues to test and re-test children for giftedness, more and more children in the community will be identified as gifted. Some researchers estimate that more than 30 kinds of bias exist. Definitions are not firm and people seem to classify almost any problem in relation to collection and analysis of information as a bias. Examples of bias present in the literature are recall, misclassification, geography, observer, lead time, over-diagnosis, length of time, response, selection, and local literature bias.

A cohort study would be a more reasonable approach to answering the spousal question than a randomized controlled trial, especially if some of the analyses could use already-collected data such as national census data or health data from those countries that have socialized health care systems.

The results of cohort studies, as for randomized controlled trial studies of etiology questions, are presented as **relative risks (RR)** with **confidence intervals (CIs)**: a statistical approximation of the increased risk for the outcome that the exposure studied conferred on the study participants. (See the end of this section for a fuller definition and an example of a calculation of relative risk.) Relative risk is the measure of the risk that one will develop the outcome (increased or decreased risk of dying) if one has the exposure of high income or low job status compared with not having the exposure.

Case-Control Studies

The **case-control study** is a less powerful methodology than the randomized controlled trial and the cohort study. Researchers conducting case-control studies select people with and without the outcome of interest and then go back in time to assess their exposure. Researchers take persons with the disease or condition (spousal socioeconomic situation) or other outcome of interest (mortality and the age when the death occurred) and match each spouse who has died with another person who is alive. Often, pairing of the people is done to have the groups (dead or alive) be similar in other features or confounding factors.

For each member of these pairs, the researchers check back in time for the presence or absence of the causative agent (education, job status, and income). In our example of spousal affect on mortality, the investigators would "pair" each spouse who had died (case) with another person of the same gender who is still alive (control). Researchers would then analyze how many of the "cases" and "controls" have had the various exposures by using existing data or interviews with individuals and family members. If more people with higher education died earlier, one could conclude that an association may exist between spousal education and mortality.

The results of case-control studies are presented as **odds ratios (OR)**. (See the end of this section for definition and calculation.) The OR is a measure of the likelihood that one was exposed to the risk factor (e.g., spouse with higher education) now that one has the outcome (e.g., one's own later or earlier death).

The case-control study design is considered "weak," or at least weaker than some designs, because exposure data are usually collected by asking people to remember and report on exposures that happened many years before. Often the best thing that can be said about human memory is that it is selective. An example of where reporting of previous exposures can be biased is in the question of whether breastfeeding (exposure) is protective against breast cancer (the disease outcome). In a case-control study, women with breast cancer may remember and report their history of breastfeeding differently than women who do not have breast cancer. Another example of where remembering exposures can be problematic is a study of the long-term consequences of using aluminum pots and pans for everyday cooking. Some research shows that aluminum exposure increases the risk for development of Alzheimer disease. In a case-control study, asking men and women with Alzheimer disease to report the constitution of their pots and pans over the past 50 to 60 years might not be the best way to collect data to answer that question.

A case-control study might provide data to answer the question of spousal effects on mortality. Again data could come from national or regional statistics and national health statistics. However, if the same data could feed both studies, the cohort study would provide the stronger evidence.

Cross-Sectional Studies with Statistically Adjusted Groups

Cross-sectional studies that use statistical adjustment of groups can also be used to compare one group of persons with another and make deductions about cause and effect. Many truths have first been recognized using this kind of research; however, many misrepresentations have also occurred. Examples are numerous in the literature for both truth finding and confusion. Using cross-sectional studies to answer our question about spouse characteristics and mortality, the researchers would have taken a group of spouses, some of whom had living partners and some whose partners had died, and compare educational levels, job status, and income of the spouses—the exposures. These exposures would then be analyzed to determine if they were related to the mortality of the partners. In many cross-sectional studies, groups are often formed by using convenience samples obtained from shopping malls, workplaces, nursing homes, universities, or other locations. Researchers rely on statisticians to adjust the findings from the groups to correct or balance for bias, confounders, and problems associated with the cross-sectional research methodology.

The biggest methodology problem associated with cross-sectional studies is that both the exposure and the outcomes are assessed at the same time, and no one can tell which came first. For example, a cross-sectional study would not be able to assess if depression caused men to be overweight or being overweight caused men to be depressed: the cross-sectional study could only measure the rates of being depressed and being overweight in a group of people. A cross-sectional study could provide evidence on our question but this evidence would not be strong—it would at best be suggestive to continue the research using stronger methods.

Resolution: Do Spousal Characteristics Affect Mortality?

Skalicka and Kunst[1] studied the education, job status, and income of spouses in Norway and determined all-cause mortality and mortality from cardiovascular disease, ischemic hart disease, stroke, all cancers, lung cancer, breast cancer, and prostate cancer for their partners. They use a cohort study of 74,599 adults living in central Norway during 1984 to 1986. Most of the couples in the region were enrolled (88% of the population) and were followed until the end of 2003 (average of 19 to 21 years of follow-up). This study evaluated 18,100 married women and 23,046 married men. Education was classified into 4 levels: primary education (9 years or less), lower secondary (10-11 years), upper secondary (12 years), and tertiary education (at least 13 years). Their present (2003) or last held occupation was taken as their profession throughout the study. Profession was classified into 7 categories from upper class through to lower class and not working. Income was categorized into 4 quartiles using all incomes in the region taken from national statistics. Men had higher incomes and more education than the women. The data were adjusted to take into account the ages of the people when they entered the study (age-adjusted data).

For women, some data suggested a slight decrease in mortality based on the husbands' higher income, educational level, and occupational status.

For men, however the data showed more and stronger evidence of spousal effect on their mortality. For example, a primary-school educated wife increased the husband's risk of dying by 26% (hazards ratio [HR] 1.26; 95% CI 1.06 to 1.51). For cause-specific mortality in women, the husband's higher class occupation was associated with 41% decreased ischemic heart disease mortality, his increased income with 81% decreased stroke mortality, and his higher education with 31% less cardiovascular mortality. For men, the wife's higher education reduced his mortality from ischemic heart disease by 80% and cardiovascular mortality by 69%. These data on cause-specific mortality are fully adjusted using the ages of the people at baseline and all of both partners' socioeconomic position data.

These data on spousal socioeconomic effects on mortality came from a strong cohort study and can likely be believed. Transferring the knowledge gained, however, means that we have to extrapolate from Norwegian married couples to our own situation. We can probably say, however, that men who marry librarians or health care professionals have made a good choice if they are interested in a long life.

COMPARISON OF DESIGNS

In summary, the cross-sectional studies with statistically adjusted groups are the easiest to complete, and are a fast way to do etiology research. Most clinicians and researchers, however, do not consider such studies to be valid enough to use in making informed health care decisions, especially if studies with stronger methods exist that have different conclusions. These cross-sectional studies are often used for an initial, quick check on an idea (e.g., does an association exist between doing crossword puzzles in hospital wards and early discharge?).

Case-control studies are marginally harder to do than cross-sectional studies, and may take a little more time, but they produce evidence that is somewhat stronger. Even though case-control studies are considered to have relatively weak methodology, they have a place in health care research. Case-control studies can be used to study rare side effects of treatments, because researchers do not need to assemble a large number of study participants and then wait for the events to occur—the events have already taken place. Case-control studies can be done relatively quickly, because the researchers do not have to wait until the disease or condition develops: the disease is already present, and only the exposures from the past need to be assessed. Doll and Hill produced the first case-control study and showed an incredibly strong association between tobacco smoking and lung cancer.[2] The associations between toxic shock syndrome and tampon use[3] and between Reye syndrome and aspirin use in children[4] were both shown in well-done case-control studies, as well as some of the first HIV studies in gay communities. The strengths of association were so strong in these studies that they far outweighed potential problems with the weaker methods. Because the studies could be done in a short period of time once researchers came to suspect the associations, knowledge gains were made quickly, lives were saved, suffering alleviated, and research agendas advanced.

Cohort studies are harder to do, and take even more time to complete, than case-control studies: In cohort studies groups are formed based on the exposures or risk factors, and the disease or other outcomes will develop in the future. Cohort studies have a stronger methodology and are prone to fewer biases than case-control studies, and therefore their evidence is considered stronger than that of case-control studies when making clinical decisions. Randomized controlled trials have both the strongest methodology and the strongest evidence, but they are difficult, if not impossible, to do to answer etiology questions.

ISSUES

Ethics and Logistics

Several issues provide challenges in conducting etiology/harm studies. **Ethics** is probably one of the most challenging issues. The strongest evidence comes from studies where researchers control who gets which exposures. However, researchers cannot control each person's exposures or risk factors for diseases and conditions. One cannot purposely expose people to things like divorce, poverty, poor eating habits, obesity and so on. To get around the issue of assigning people to potentially troubling exposures or unrealistic positive exposures such as high salaries or advanced education, researchers move to observing those people who already have these conditions or exposures—weaker evidence. Ethics also comes into play here as identifying and following people with exposures such as incest or addictive behaviors cause discomfort and give rise to ethical challenges.

Logistics also play a major role in the design of high-quality etiology studies because of the difficulty of controlling or even understanding exposures, such as living next to factories or electric power lines, and the length of time it takes for such diseases as leukemia or other conditions to develop. For example, some endocrinologists feel that early exposure to cow's milk is a risk factor for a child to develop diabetes mellitus in later life. To assess this, a randomized controlled trial is probably not feasible, because few mothers would consent to being randomized to either breastfeed their children or use cow's milk for their newborn infants. Some research already shows that cow's milk is not good for infants less than 1 year old because of allergies and nutritional and other problems. A cohort design can present similar problems with the exposures. However, a study of children, some of whom are breastfed and some of whom are given cow's milk, would need to follow all of the children for at least 20 years to be able to assess the rates of development of adult-onset diabetes. A case-control study or a study with a cross-sectional design with statistically adjusted groups may be the only possible alternative to evaluate the question of an association between early cow's milk exposure and development of diabetes mellitus during adulthood.

Blinding

From a methodological point of view, **blinding** is probably the most important issue in causation studies. Blinding is slightly more important for those studies with weaker methodologies: case-control studies and cross-sectional studies with statistically adjusted groups. All study designs must assess both exposures and outcomes, but this assessment is done at different times for each of the 4 study types. Exposure is assessed in the future for randomized controlled trials, in the present for many cohort studies, and in the past for case-control studies and cross-sectional studies with statistically adjusted groups. The people who assess the exposures (e.g., high IQ) must be blinded to the outcomes (e.g., high income at age 40) *and* the persons who assess the outcomes (e.g., high income at age 40) must be blinded to the exposures (e.g., high IQ) in a study determining if intelligence contributes to high salaries. Blinding is less important when the outcomes are objective. This means that if the outcome for an etiology study is all-cause mortality, the blinding is not as important—a death is a death, is a death. No blinding statement was observed in the study of spousal characteristics and all-cause and cause-specific mortality.[1] Other examples of objective outcomes are confirmed divorces, birthweight, or a laboratory confirmed diagnosis when the laboratory output is taken from a machine and involves little chance for misreading the results. Although blinding is often crucial for etiology/causation studies, it is not often indexed by MEDLINE.

Association versus Causation

Another important issue in understanding etiology is that, just because 2 things occur at the same time (are associated), one does not necessarily cause the other. As a rather extreme example, the rate of influenza is lower in the summer than in the winter. People also eat more ice cream in the summer. No one would, however, link eating ice cream with a decreased risk for the flu. Health care personnel regularly struggle with the issue of association not being the same as causation. One example of this is a series of Finnish studies by Salonen et al.[5] In 1992 they reported that persons who had a myocardial infarction also had high levels of stored iron in their blood. The only effective, low-cost clinical method of reducing iron levels is extracting blood from the individuals. Some blood donor organizations, using these association data, developed an advertising program that encouraged persons to donate blood to reduce their risk for having a myocardial infarction.

Not all researchers or clinicians believe that the iron levels-and-heart attack association is true. They feel that the association found by Salonen et al has not been proved with sufficient strength of evidence that such decisions as the development and use of aggressive advertising programs to increase blood donor response are justified. Etiology studies must be assessed carefully, and common sense must be applied in understanding and using them for clinical decisions.

HOW RESULTS OF ETIOLOGY STUDIES ARE REPORTED

Relative Risk

Both relative risks (RR) and odds ratios (OR) are used to statistically represent the associations found in etiology studies. **Relative risk** is the risk or rate of developing a disease in the exposed group divided by the risk or rate of developing the disease in those who were not exposed. Cohort studies and randomized controlled trials present their findings using RR. An example of using RR to present data comes from the Nurses' Health Study.[6] Willett et al found that women who had gained at least 20 to 25 pounds since they were 18 years old had a lifetime RR for developing coronary heart disease of 1.90. This means that women who had gained 20 to 25 or more pounds had 90% more risk for developing coronary artery disease than women who had gained little or no weight beyond their teenage weight: basically, double the rate. Using hypothetical data we can see how this RR of 1.9 was calculated.

Of 200 women with a weight gain of at least 20 to 25 pounds since adolescence, 106 women developed coronary artery disease during their lifetimes. This risk or rate of coronary artery disease for the women who gained weight is calculated using the data: 106/200, which is 53%.

In 200 women with long-term stable weight, only 58 developed coronary heart disease. Their risk or rate for coronary artery disease is calculated as 58/200, or 26%.

To calculate the RR, we take the 2 risks from the groups and form a ratio: the rate in women with exposure (weight gain) divided by the rate in women without exposure (little or no weight gain). The calculation for the RR is thus 53%/26%, or 1.9. When the RR is greater than 1 we know that the risk is increased—more risk of the outcome for the people who are represented in the numerator of the calculation. An RR less than 1 is protective—less risk of the outcome for the people whose data are in the numerator.

Odds Ratios

Odds ratios (OR) are used to report findings from case-control studies—and in many other study designs. An OR is the ratio of the rate among people who have a disease of having been exposed in the past compared to the rate of exposure in the past among people who do not have the disease. For example, DiFranza and Lew[7] report that children who were hospitalized for lower respiratory infections have an OR of 3.3 for being exposed to parental tobacco smoke. This means that children who were hospitalized with lower respiratory infections were 3.3 times more likely to have been exposed to parental tobacco smoke than their peers who were hospitalized with a condition other than lower respiratory infections.

SUMMARY

The important issues in etiology/causation studies follow in more or less order of importance.

- Similarity of clearly identified comparison groups with respect to important determinants of outcome
- Outcomes and exposures measurements done in the same way in the groups being compared. Two-way blinding is important here: Outcome assessors should not know the exposures and those who assess the exposures should not know the outcomes
- Follow-up of sufficient length in relation to the outcomes
- Assessment of a temporal relationship (e.g., did people smoke before they got lung cancer?)
- A dose-response gradient (e.g., did heavier smokers get lung cancer sooner or at a higher rate? was the disease more severe?)
- The strength of the association between exposure and outcome
- The precision of the estimate of risk

SEARCHING METHODOLOGY

Indexers often recognize the study methodology for randomized controlled trials, cohort studies, case-control studies, and cross-sectional studies with statistically adjusted groups. In addition they index for risk in various forms and ORs. Indexers, however, use risk only for the increase in probability of the disease or condition (e.g., a family history of colorectal cancer increases one's own risk for colorectal cancer). For the "protective" effects (e.g., continued and ongoing mental stimulation may reduce the risk for Alzheimer disease), the indexers use subheadings and indexing related to prevention and control. Possible indexing terms and phrases for all 4 databases are on the following pages. Textwords are similar across all of the databases.

MEDLINE

MeSH, Subheadings, Publicaton Types, and Textwords

MeSH (Medical Subject Headings — Index Terms)

Cohort studies* (can be exploded)
Mortality*
Risk*

Age factors (can be exploded)
Age of onset
Association (can be exploded)
Bias (epidemiology) (can be exploded)
Case-control studies
Case-control studies (can be exploded)
Causality (can be exploded)
Cohort effect
Confidence intervals
Confounding factors (epidemiology)
Cross-sectional studies
Drug toxicity (can be exploded)
Effect modifiers (can be exploded)
Environmental exposure (can be exploded)
Environmental monitoring
Epidemiologic factors (can be exploded)
Epidemiologic studies (can be exploded)
Follow-up studies
Incidence
Inhalation exposure
Logistic models
Longitudinal studies (can be exploded)
Matched-pair analysis
Maternal exposure
Maximum allowable concentration
Morbidity (can be exploded)
Observer variation
Occupational exposure (can be exploded)
Odds ratio
Paternal exposure
Poverty (can be exploded)
Precipitating factors

---

*Indicates a preferred term as determined in the Clinical Hedges Study.[8]

Prevalence
Proportional hazards models
Prospective studies
Reproductive history (can be exploded)
Retrospective studies
Risk adjustment
Risk assessment (can be exploded)
Risk factors
Seroepidemiologic studies (can be exploded)
Sex factors
Social class (can be exploded)
Socioeconomic factors (can be exploded)

Subheadings

Adverse effects (can be exploded)
Chemically induced
Epidemiology (can be exploded)
Epidemiology (for distributions, causes, and attributes of disease)
Etiology
Genetic
Poisoning
Prevention and control
Toxicity

Publication Types

None

Textwords (Same List Is Used for All 4 Databases)

Between group*
Cohort*
Cohort study*
Mortal:*
Mortality*
Randomized*
Relative risk*
Risk*
Risk factor*

Absolute risk increas:
Absolute risk reduct:
Absolute risk:
Adjusted odds ratio:

---

*Indicates a preferred term as determined in the Clinical Hedges Study.[8-10]

Adjusted OR
Advers: drug reaction:
Advers: effect:
Advers: event:
Adverse drug reaction:
Adverse effect:
Adverse event:
Adverse outcome:
Aetiological stud:
Aetiology
Analytic stud:
Analytical stud:
ARI
ARR
Associate:
Association
Attributable risk:
Blind:
Case comparison:
Case control:
Case referent stud:
Case referent:
Case series
Case-control stud:
Caus:
Causal
Causal agent:
Causal analys:
Causality
Causation
Cause-and-effect
Cause-and-effect hypothes:
Cause-and-effect relation:
Cause:
CI
Cofactor:
Cohort analys:
Cohort analytic stud:
Cohort stud:
Comparison group:
Comparison:
Complication:
Concurrent cohort stud:
Confidence interval:
Cross-sectional stud:

Disease risk:
Dose-response curve:
Dose-response relation:
Dose-response relationship:
Dose-response:
Etiolog:
Etiological stud:
Exposure group:
Exposure:
Follow-up stud:
Follow-up:
Follow-up: period:
Follow-up: stud:
Harm:
Harmful agent:
Harmful outcome:
Hazard ratio:
Hazard:
Historical cohort stud:
HR
Incidence
Incidence rate:
Longitudinal stud:
Multicausal
Multiple causation
Negative outcome:
Nested case-control stud:
Nested case-control:
NNH
Number needed to harm
Numbers needed to harm
Observational stud:
Odds ratio:
OR
Population attributable fraction:
Population attributable risk:
Precipitation factor:
Prospective cohort stud:
Prospective stud:
Rate ratio:
Referent
Relation
Relative frequenc:
Relative hazard:
Retrospective stud:

Risk assessment:
Risk cofactor:
Risk difference:
Risk probabilit:
Risk ratio:
RR
Side effect:
Temporal relation:
Toxic:
Toxicit:

CINAHL (CUMULATIVE INDEX TO NURSING AND ALLIED HEALTH LITERATURE)

Index Terms, Subheadings, and Publication Types

Index Terms

Relative risk*
Survival analysis*
Treatment outcomes*

Age factors
Age of onset
Analytic research
Cardiovascular risk factors
Case control studies (can be exploded)
Concurrent prospective studies
Confidence intervals
Correlational studies
Cox proportional hazards model
Cross sectional studies
Drug toxicity (can be exploded)
Environmental exposure (can be exploded)
Environmental monitoring (can be exploded)
Epidemiological research (can be exploded)
Hospital-based case control
Incidence
Matched case control
Maternal exposure
Medical, evidence based
Morbidity (can be exploded)
Nonconcurrent prospective studies
Nonexperimental studies (can be exploded)

*Indicates a preferred term as determined in the Clinical Hedges Study.[9]

Nursing practice, evidence based
Occupational exposure
Occupational therapy, evidence based
Odds ratio
Organizations (can be exploded)
Panel studies
Physiotherapy, evidence based
Population-based case control
Poverty (can be exploded)
Prevalence
Professional practice, evidence based
Professional practice, research based (can be exploded)
Prospective studies (can be exploded)
Pseudolongitudinal studies
Reproductive history
Research (can be exploded)
Retrospective design
Retrospective panel studies
Retrospective studies
Revolving panel studies
Risk assessment
Risk factors (can be exploded)
Seroprevalence studies
Sex factors
Social class (can be exploded)
Socioeconomic factors (can be exploded)
Toxic inhalation (can be exploded)

Subheadings

Adverse effects
Chemically induced
Epidemiology
Etiology
Familial and genetic
Nursing (also gets lots of therapy and diagnosis studies)
Poisoning
Prevention and control

Publication Types

Clinical trial*

Research

---

*Indicates a preferred term as determined in the Clinical Hedges Study.[9]

EMBASE

Index Terms, Subheadings, and Publication Types

Index Terms

Methodology* (can be exploded)
Epidemiology* (can be exploded)
Risk factor

Adverse drug reaction (can be exploded)
Analytic method
Anamnesis (can be exploded)
Association
Attributable risk
Cancer risk
Cardiovascular risk
Case control study
Case study
Cause of death
Cohort analysis
Comparative study (can be exploded)
Complication (can be exploded)
Coronary risk
Correlational Study
Cross Sectional Study
Dose response (can be exploded)
Drug toxicity (can be exploded)
Environmental exposure
Environmental monitoring (can be exploded)
Epidemiology (can be exploded)
Etiology (can be exploded)
Exposure
Exposure (can be exploded)
Fetus risk
Follow up
Genetic risk
Hazard (can be exploded)
Health hazard (can be exploded)
High risk behavior
High risk patient
High risk population
High risk pregnancy

*Indicates a preferred term as determined in the Clinical Hedges Study.[10]

Hospital-based case control study
Incidence (can be exploded)
Infection risk
Longitudinal study
Maximum allowable concentration
Morbidity (can be exploded)
Nonbiological model (can be exploded)
Observer variation
Occupational exposure
Occupational health (can be exploded)
Onset age
Population Risk
Population-based case control study
Poverty
Prevalence (can be exploded)
Prospective study
Recurrence risk
Retrospective study
Risk (can be exploded)
Risk assessment
Risk benefit analysis
Risk factor
Risk management
Risk reduction
Sex difference
Side effect (can be exploded)
Social class
Social status (can be exploded)
Socioeconomic (can be exploded)
Statistical analysis (can be exploded)
Statistical model
Statistics (can be exploded)
Toxicity (can be exploded)

Subheadings

Adverse drug reactions
Complication
Congenital disorder
Drug interaction
Drug toxicity
Epidemiology
Etiology
Heredity

Side effect
Toxicity

Publication Types

Adverse drug reactions
Etiology
Fatality
Iatrogenic disease
Intoxication
Congenital disorder
Prevention
Side effects
Drug toxicity

PsycINFO

Index Terms, Subheadings, and Publication Types

Index Terms

At risk populations
Attribution
Causal analysis
Causality
Cohort analysis
Confidence limits, statistics
Coronary prone behavior
Disadvantaged
Drug induced congenital disorder (can be exploded)
Environmental effects
Epidemiology
Etiology
Experimenter bias
Followup studies
Human sex differences
Income level (can be exploded)
Longitudinal studies (can be exploded)
Obstetrical complications
Occupational exposure
Onset disorders
Postsurgical complications
Poverty
Predisposition
Premorbidity

Prenatal exposure
Prevention (can be exploded)
Prospective studies
Protective factors
Psychosocial factors
Racial and ethnic differences
Retrospective studies
Risk analysis
Risk factors
Side effects, drug (can be exploded)
Side effects, treatment (can be exploded)
Social class (can be exploded)
Social deprivation (can be exploded)
Social issues (can be exploded)
Sociocultural factors (can be exploded)
Socioeconomic status (can be exploded)
Susceptibility disorders
Teratogens
Toxicity

Subheadings

Between Groups Design
Causal Analysis
Cohort Analysis
Cohort Analysis
Empirical Methods (can be exploded)
Experiment Controls (used for control groups)
Experiment Volunteers (can be exploded)
Experimental Methods
Experimental Subjects
Follow-up Studies
Longitudinal Studies
Observation Methods
Prospective Studies
Repeated Measures
Retrospective Studies

Publication Types

Empirical Study
Follow-up Study
Longitudinal Study
Prospective Study
Retrospective Study

EXAMPLES OF TEXTWORDS AND INDEXING USING OUR CLINICAL EXAMPLE

Citation for Our Clinical Example

Baker DW, Wolf MS, Feinglass J, Thompson JA. Health literacy, cognitive abilities, and mortality among elderly persons. J Gen Intern Med. 2008 Jun;23(6):723-6.

Textwords and Index Terms Used in Our Clinical Example

Textwords (in the Title and Abstract of the Article)

Prospective cohort study
All-cause mortality
Cause-specific mortality
Crude mortality rates
Adjusting for demographics, socioeconomic status and baseline health
Hazards ratios
Multivariate models
Risk-adjusted rates

MEDLINE INDEXING

Mortality (subheading)
Prospective studies
Proportional hazards model

CIHAHL INDEXING

Mortality (subheading)
Cox proportional hazards model
Mortality
Prospective studies

EMBASE INDEXING

Cohort analysis
Multivariate analysis
Prospective study

PROVEN STRATEGIES

Search Strategies (Filters) Derived during the Clinical Hedges Study[8-10]

Filter*	MEDLINE	CINAHL†	EMBASE
Sensitive	risk:.mp. OR exp cohort studies OR between group:.tw.	randomized.tw. OR treatment outcomes.sh. OR clinical trial.pt.	risk:.mp. OR exp methodology OR exp epidemiology
Specific	relative risk:.tw. OR risks.tw. OR cohort stud:.mp.	exp survival analysis OR relative risk.mp.	cohort.tw. OR relative risk:.tw.
Maximize difference between Sensitivity and Specificity	risk.mp. OR mortality.mp. OR cohort.tw.	confidence interval:.mp. OR mortalit:.mp. OR risk factor:.mp.	risk.tw. OR mortalit:.tw. OR cohort.tw.

*See the Introduction for a description of how to use these filters and where to find them in Ovid and PubMed.
†In 2009, CINAHL will only be offered through EBSCO. The CINAHL search strategies have been translated and are available for use in EBSCO.

EXERCISES

Note that the search possibilities (answers) are detailed in the Appendix.

1. Alzheimer disease is becoming more common—maybe because the baby boomers are getting older. Find all the risk factors you can—factors that are protective and those associated with an increased risk. Grade the evidence you find according to the following categories:

   - Grade A Randomized controlled trials
   - Grade B Cohort studies
   - Grade C Case-control studies
   - Grade D Case series (5 to 20 patients and no control group)
   - Grade E Case reports (1 or 2 persons) and opinion

2. Health literacy seems to be an important topic. Does evidence exist that good health literacy is associated with improved mortality?

REFERENCES

1. Skalicka V, Kunst AE. Effects of spouses' socioeconomic characteristics on mortality among men and women in a Norwegian longitudinal study. *Soc Sci Med.* 2008;66:2035-2047.

2. Doll R, Hill AB. Smoking and carcinoma of the lung: preliminary report. 1950. *Br Med J.* 1950;2:739-748.

3. Shands KN, Schmid GP, Dan BB, et al. Toxic-shock syndrome in menstruating women: association with tampon use and *Staphylococcus aureus* and clinical features in 52 cases. *N Engl J Med.* 1980;303:1436-1442.

4. Hurwitz ES, Barrett MJ, Bregman D, et al. Public Health Service study of Reye's syndrome and medications. Report of the main study. *JAMA.* 1987;257:1905-1911.

5. Salonen JT, Nyyssonen K, Korpela H, et al. High stored iron levels are associated with excess risk of myocardial infarction in eastern Finnish men. *Circulation.* 1992;86:803-811.

6. Willett WC, Manson JE, Stampfer MJ, et al. Weight, weight change, and coronary heart disease in women. Risk within the "normal" weight range. *JAMA.* 1995;273:461-465.

7. DiFranza JR, Lew RA. Morbidity and mortality in children associated with the use of tobacco products by other people. *Pediatrics.* 1996;97:560-568.

8. Wilczynski NL, Haynes RB; Hedges Team. Developing optimal search strategies for detecting clinically sound causation studies in MEDLINE. *AMIA Annu Symp Proc.* 2003:719-723.

9. Walker-Dilks C, Wilczynski NL, Haynes RB; Hedges Team. Cumulative Index to Nursing and Allied Health Literature search strategies for identifying methodologically sound causation and prognosis studies. *Appl Nurs Res.* 2008;21:98-103.

10. Haynes RB, Kastner M, Wilczynski NL; Hedges Team. Developing optimal search strategies for detecting clinically sound and relevant causation studies in EMBASE. *BMC Med Inform Decis Mak.* 2005;5:8

5

Natural History and Prognosis

Nancy Wilczynski

INTRODUCTION

Another type of primary clinical research we will now look at has 2 designations: natural history and prognosis. Traditionally, **natural history** has been considered the progression of untreated disease, and **prognosis** is the progression of treated disease. A more recent definition has natural history starting earlier in the disease process—at the time that changes start to happen at the cellular level in humans; prognosis starts after the disease has been diagnosed. Health care professionals must have ready access to natural history and prognosis information to respond to their patients' requests. One of the first questions patients ask when they are given a new diagnosis is "what will happen to me now?" They want to know the implications of their newly diagnosed disease or condition for survival, disease progression, and lifestyle, even before they start to assess treatment or palliative care options and issues. Some epidemiologists consider that the major issue for natural history and prognosis studies is *whether* to treat. This is in contrast with therapy, where the issue is *how* to treat; with diagnosis, where the issue is *what* to treat; and with etiology, where the issue is *how did I get here*?

A high-quality prognosis and natural history study is done using a cohort study design. A group of people with a specific disease are followed over time to discover their disease progression. The patients are often newly diagnosed or at an early stage; having a high follow-up rate is important for study quality and validity of the study results.

CLINICAL EXAMPLE

Once again, as with the previous chapters, we will start with an example of a problem and the research that went into solving it. The problem was that there was little consistency and a great deal of variation in the survival times reported for patient with dementia. Additionally, there was considerable uncertainty about what factors influenced survival in patients with dementia. Xie and colleagues[1] conducted a study to provide estimates of survival after the onset of dementia, taking into account the patient's age, sex, self-reported health, disability, and severity of cognitive impairment. They studied 438 participants who developed dementia from a population based study of 13,004 individuals aged 65 years and older. Participants were interviewed over a 10-year period and were followed for 14 years to determine if they had died. Individuals with prevalent dementia (i.e., existing dementia) at the time of entry into the cohort were excluded from the analyses; thus, an inception cohort (defined later in the chapter) was assembled. By December 2005, 356 of the 438 (81%) participants who had developed dementia had died. Median survival time from onset of dementia to death was 4.1 years for men and 4.6 years for women. There was a difference of nearly 7 years in survival between the younger old and the oldest people with dementia: 10.7 years for ages 65-69 years; 5.4 for ages 70-79; 4.3 for ages 80-89, and 3.8 years for ages ≥90.

To determine which factors were predictive of mortality, the authors used Cox's proportional hazards regression models and reported hazard ratios. A hazard ratio in a survival analysis is the effect of an explanatory factor (e.g., sex) on the hazard or risk of an event (e.g., death). The authors found that sex, age of onset, and disability were statistically predictive of mortality in the presence of dementia. They concluded that the results of this study could be used to provide prognostic information to individuals as well as for planning for patients, care givers, service providers, and policy makers.

HOW NATURAL HISTORY AND PROGNOSIS STUDIES ARE DONE

All patients, regardless of their disease, want to know the implications of their disease. Some diseases and conditions do not require treatment, or current treatments have not proved beneficial (e.g., the common cold). Some diseases and conditions need immediate, active treatment (e.g., major hemorrhage, peptic ulcers, myocardial infarction, and appendicitis). For some, if not all, diseases, it is important for the patient and health care professional to come to a decision on whether to pursue treatment. A classic and important example that demands balance between the disease progression characteristics and treatment options is the child with a slight-to-moderate degree of scoliosis (curvature of the spine). Children with scoliosis can be crippled or even die if they are not treated in an appropriate and timely manner. Several effective therapies exist, but they are unpleasant and invasive, involving surgery and long-term body casts. Not all children with scoliosis, however, need treatment. Good prognostic information exists to help clinicians, patients, and families make wise decisions on a case-by-case basis.

NATURAL HISTORY VERSUS PROGNOSIS

Natural history and prognosis, although related, are not equivalent concepts. To reiterate, natural history has traditionally been considered to follow untreated disease to see what happens over time. Probably the best-known natural history study is the Tuskegee Study of Untreated Syphilis in the Negro Male.[2] The study commenced in 1931, and enrolled 399 African American men with tertiary syphilis and 201 uninfected men, and followed them while withholding treatment until 1972. Of course, this study was obviously unethical and should never have been done. Allowing untreated disease to progress when even marginally effective treatments are available is unacceptable: Science must never be allowed to come before ethics, human dignity, and common sense.

Prognosis, on the other hand, has traditionally been considered the study of treated disease over time. For example, stroke is a common disease that is treated in the hospital and at home with a variety of medical, nursing, physiotherapeutic, occupational therapy, and at times, psychological interventions. The Oxfordshire Community Stroke Project study[3] is a good example of a prognosis study in this population. The study assessed outcomes after a first-ever stroke in 675 patients who were followed for up to 6.5 years. The Oxfordshire data showed that mortality after stroke was 19% in the first 30 days and 31% in the first year. For those people who survived beyond the first year, mortality in the subsequent years decreased substantially.

The more current distinction between natural history and prognosis is that *natural history* starts at the biologic onset of disease and includes the periods when early diagnosis (with no symptoms) is possible, through to the time when usual clinical diagnosis occurs and to final outcome assessment. This is a 4-stage process, with the first stage being very difficult to ascertain, if not impossible, to realize. *Prognosis* includes the time from clinical diagnosis through to outcome assessment (the 2 final stages of natural history). A natural history study of myocardial infarction, for example, would start with the development of atherosclerosis; a prognosis study would start at the onset of chest pain.

INCEPTION COHORT STUDIES

The key issue in studying the natural history and prognosis of diseases is the collection of a *representative* sample of patients who are at an *early* stage in their disease process. Researchers assess these patients over time. This type of study design is called an **inception cohort**. "Inception" means an early, uniformed point in time for the disease; "cohort" means following a group of people forward in time—just as it did for the etiology and causation studies described in Chapter 4. When studying natural history or prognosis, it is important to identify and include patients as near to the onset of the disease as possible. This is especially true for diseases that have serious outcomes near the onset, such as stroke and bacterial meningitis. As another example, people with a myocardial infarction can die within minutes, so that studying prognosis in these patients needs to start as early as possible—probably at the front door of the emergency room, if not in the ambulance, with a check at the coroner's office for sudden deaths. Starting in the coronary care unit or a step-down unit would not truly reflect the important considerations that need to be addressed when studying the myocardial infarction disease process because many patients die before reaching these units.

Completeness of follow-up is also important for natural history and prognosis studies, as it is for therapy studies because "missing" persons can obscure the disease process. For example, a study of the progression of rheumatoid arthritis in patients who were newly diagnosed and followed in a tertiary care clinic might lose patients who had little or no disease progression. In other words, following only those patients who returned for follow-up of their rheumatoid arthritis would tend to overestimate the morbidity associated with the disease. In contrast, a study of men with advanced prostate cancer that did not include an aggressive follow-up process might "lose" men who had died. This loss to follow-up would tend to show that the prognosis of prostate cancer was better than it truly is. Again, 80% is the "magic" number for follow-up that is assumed for good quality natural history and prognosis studies. Higher levels are desirable, and lower levels of follow-up rates are unacceptable.

Length of follow-up is also important and should be judged using common sense. A prognosis study of influenza or the common cold would provide most of its useful information by 6 months to 1 year. A prognosis study of multiple sclerosis or rheumatoid arthritis needs a much longer length of follow-up—perhaps even in the range of decades.

Treatment studies using a randomized controlled trial design are another category of research that can also give good, reliable prognosis information, especially for diseases with specific treatments such as congestive heart failure. They can provide survival rates and disease progression data for the study groups or the placebo groups. Researchers need to recognize this source of information for comprehensive searching on prognosis topics.

CALCULATIONS

No special calculations or statistics are involved in natural history or prognosis studies. Quite often the reported data are similar to etiology and causation statistics and data presentation, with rates for disease progression and specific outcomes, and the risk for these outcomes, reported. For example, Prencipe and colleagues[4] reported on 322 adults who had had a minor stroke and were followed for 10 years. Ninety-six deaths occurred, along with 69 new cerebrovascular events. Hazard ratios showed that a previous myocardial infarction increased risk of dying by 1.8 times (hazard ratio 1.8; 95% CI 1.1 to 3.1).

Terminology between prognostic studies and etiologic studies may differ slightly, however. Etiology studies use the phrase risk factors—those things that increase or decrease the chance of developing a disease or disorder. For prognostic studies, the similar factor is often called a *prognostic factor*—the feature that is associated with disease progression.

SUMMARY

In summary, natural history and prognosis studies are done using an inception cohort design. Patients with a specific disease or condition are identified at diagnosis, soon after diagnosis, or at a uniform, early time in the disease process, and followed for an appropriate period of time in relation to that disease's process. A high follow-up rate (>80% is essential) is important. The Evidence-Based Medicine Working Group, in their *Users' Guides to the Literature*, outlines the attributes of natural history and prognosis studies that are of importance for clinicians [5]

- Well-defined representative sample of patients at a similar point in the course of the disease
- Length and completeness of follow-up
- Objective and unbiased outcomes criteria
- Adjustment for important prognostic factors

SEARCHING METHODOLOGY

Now that we have summarized the components of prognosis studies we move onto searching for prognostic studies in large electronic databases such as MEDLINE. This task can be challenging but using search terms that target the methodology specific to prognosis studies in addition to content terms (e.g., dementia) can aid in retrieval effectiveness. The search terms available to use in 4 of the large electronic databases follow. The terms were compiled during the Clinical Hedges Study [6] after seeking input from clinicians and librarians in the United States and Canada. Index terms, subheadings, and publication types are assigned to each article in the database by staff working for the electronic database (eg, MEDLINE). Textwords are used to search for articles using the article title and the article abstract. Preferred search terms are shown for MEDLINE, EMBASE, and CINAHL as search strategies were developed for detecting prognostic studies during the Clinical Hedges Study for these 3 databases.

MEDLINE

MeSH, Subheadings, Publication Types, and Textwords

MeSH (Medical Subject Headings—Index Terms)

Cohort studies* (can be exploded)
Epidemiologic studies (can be exploded) *
Incidence*
Models, statistical (can be exploded)*
Mortality (can be exploded) *
Follow-up studies*
Prognosis* (can be exploded)

Age factors (can be exploded)
Age of onset
Death (can be exploded)
Disease (can be exploded)
Disease-free survival
Disease progression
Hospital mortality
Infant mortality
Life expectancy
Longitudinal studies (can be exploded)
Maternal mortality
Morbidity (can be exploded)
Natural history
Prospective studies
Sex factors
Survival analysis (can be exploded)
Survival rate
Time factors

Subheadings

Epidemiology (can be exploded)
Mortality (can be exploded)

Publication Types

None

---

*Indicates a preferred term as determined in the Clinical Hedges Study.[7]

Textwords (Same List Is Used for All 4 Databases)

Cohort*
Cohort:*
Course:*
Death*
Diagnos:*
Diagnosed*
First episode*
Follow-up*
Outcome*
Predict:*
Predictor:*
Prospective stud:*
Prognos:*
Risk:*
Survival*

Adjusted hazard: ratio:
"Adjusted HR"
All-cause mortalit:
Cohort analys:
Cohort analytic stud:
Cohort stud:
Cox proportional hazard:
Cox regression
Death:
Death rate:
Disease course:
Disease onset
Disease-free survival
Disease progression
Early onset
Early stage
Epidemiologic stud:
First admission
First diagnosis
Follow-up stud:
Hazard ratio:
Hazards ratio:
HR
Hospital mortalit:

---

*Indicates a preferred term as determined in the Clinical Hedges Study.[7-9]

Inception
Inception cohort:
Inciden:
Infant mortalit:
Life expectancy
Longitudinal stud:
Maternal mortality
Morbidity
Mortality
Natural history
Predictive
Predictive factor:
Prognosis
Prognostic:
Prognostic factor:
Remission rate:
Survival analys:
Survival rate
Survival time:
Time factors
Tumor progression
Tumour progression

CINAHL (CUMULATIVE INDEX TO NURSING AND ALLIED HEALTH LITERATURE)

Index Terms, Subheadings, and Publication Types

Index Terms

Diagnosis* (can be exploded)
Economics* (can be exploded)
"Outcomes (health care)" (can be exploded)*
Study design (can be exploded)*
Prospective studies* (can be exploded)

Age factors
Age of onset
Comorbidity
Cox proportional hazards model
Critical illness
Death (can be exploded)

---

*Indicates a preferred term as determined in the Clinical Hedges Study.[8]

Disease duration
Disease progression
Disease remission
Disease (can be exploded)
Hospital mortality
Incidence
Infant mortality
Life expectancy
Maternal mortality
Morbidity (can be exploded)
Mortality (can be exploded)
Perinatal death
Predictive research
Prognosis (can be exploded)
Recovery
Recurrence
Sex factors.
Survival analysis (can be exploded)
Survival
Time factors

Subheadings

Epidemiology
Mortality

Publication Types

None

EMBASE

Index Terms, Subheadings, and Publication Types

Index Terms

Diagnosis* (can be exploded)
Disease course (can be exploded)*
Follow up*
"General aspect of disease" (can be exploded)*
"Physical disease by body function" (can be exploded)*

---

*Indicates a preferred term as determined in the Clinical Hedges Study.[9]

Risk* (can be exploded)

Cancer survival
Cancer recurrence
Cause of death
Cohort analysis
Comorbidity
Death (can be exploded)
Disease duration
Dying
Epidemiology (can be exploded)
Fatality
Fetus death (can be exploded)
Incidence (can be exploded)
Infant mortality
Life expectancy
Longitudinal study
Maternal morbidity
Morbidity (can be exploded)
Mortality (can be exploded)
Onset age
Prediction
Prognosis
Proportional hazards model
Prospective study
Recurrent disease
Relapse
Remission
Survival rate
Survival time
Survival (can be exploded)
Terminal disease
Time (can be exploded)
Treatment failure
Tumor recurrence

Subheadings

Epidemiology*

Publication Types

None

---

*Indicates a preferred term as determined in the Clinical Hedges Study.[9]

PsycINFO

Index Terms, Subheadings, and Publication Types

Index Terms

Cohort analysis
Comorbidity
"Death and dying" (can be exploded)
Disease course
Diseases
Disorders (can be exploded)
Followup studies
Life expectancy
Longitudinal studies (can be exploded)
Mortality rate
"Onset, disorders"
Prediction
Prognosis
Prospective studies
"Recovery (disorders)"
"Relapse (disorders)"
"Remission (disorders)" (can be exploded)
Spontaneous remission
Sudden infant death
Symptom remission

Subheadings

None

Publication Types

None

EXAMPLES OF TEXTWORDS AND INDEXING USING OUR CLINICAL EXAMPLE

Citation for Our Clinical Example

Xie J, Brayne C, Matthews FE; Medical Research Council Cognitive Function and Ageing Study collaborators. Survival times in people with dementia: analysis from a population based cohort study with 14 year follow-up. *BMJ.* 2008;336:258-262.

Textwords and Index Terms Used in Our Clinical Example

Textwords (in the Title and Abstract of the Article)

Cohort*
Diagnos:*
Follow-up*
Predict:*
Predictor:*
Survival*

Cohort stud:
Death
Inciden:
Mortality
Survival time:

MEDLINE INDEXING

Age of onset
Mortality (subheading)
Epidemiology (subheading)

CINAHL INDEXING

Age of onset
Mortality (subheading)

EMBASE INDEXING

Epidemiology* (subheading)
Follow up*

Cohort analysis
Death
Mortality
Onset age
Proportional hazards model
Prospective study
Survival time

---

*Indicates a preferred term as determined in the Clinical Hedges Study.[7-9]

PROVEN STRATEGIES

Search Strategies (Filters) Derived during the Clinical Hedges Study[7-9]

Filter*	MEDLINE (Ovid syntax)	CINAHL† (Ovid syntax)	EMBASE (Ovid syntax)
Sensitive	incidence.sh. OR exp mortality OR follow-up studies.sh. OR prognos:.tw. OR predict:.tw. OR course:.tw.	exp study design OR diagnos:.mp. OR outcome.mp.	exp disease course OR risk:.mp. OR diagnos:.mp. OR follow-up.mp. OR ep.fs. OR outcome.tw.
Specific	prognos:.tw. OR first episode.tw. OR cohort.tw.	prognos:.tw. OR prospective studies.sh.	prognos:.tw. OR survival.tw.
Minimize difference between Sensitivity and Specificity	prognosis.sh. OR diagnosed.tw. OR cohort:.mp. OR predictor:.tw. OR death.tw. OR exp "models, statistical"	diagnos:.tw. OR exp "outcomes (health care)" OR prospective studies.sh.	follow-up.mp. OR prognos:.tw. OR ep.fs.

*See the Introduction for a description of how to use these filters and where to find them in Ovid and PubMed.
† In 2009 CINAHL will only be offered through EBSCO. The CINAHL search strategies have been translated and are available for use in EBSCO.

LINKS TO OTHER RESOURCES

Link to information regarding the Clinical Hedges Study: http://hiru.mcmaster.ca/hiru/HIRU_McMaster_HKR.aspx

Link to How to use an article about prognosis: http://www.cche.net/usersguides/prognosis.asp

EXERCISES

Note that the search possibilities (answers) are detailed in the Appendix.

1. What is the long-term prognosis of Crohn disease?
2. Are there factors that predict survival in patients with advanced esophageal cancer?

REFERENCES

1. Xie J, Brayne C, Matthews FE; Medical Research Council Cognitive Function and Ageing Study collaborators. Survival times in people with dementia: analysis from a population based cohort study with 14 year follow-up. *BMJ.* 2008;336:258-262.

2. Brawley OW. The study of untreated syphilis in the negro male. *Int J Radiat Oncol Biol Phys.* 1998;40:5-8.

3. Dennis MS, Burn JP, Sandercock PA, et al. Long-term survival after first-ever stroke: the Oxfordshire Community Stroke Project. *Stroke.* 1993;24:796-800.

4. Prencipe M, Culasso F, Rasura M, et al. Long-term prognosis after a minor stroke. 10-year mortality and major stroke recurrence in a hospital-based cohort. *Stroke.* 1998;29:126-132.

5. Guyatt G, Rennie D, Meade MO, Cook DJ. *Users' Guide to the Medical Literature. A Manual for Evidence-Based Clinical Practice.* 2 ed. New York, NY: McGraw-Hill Companies Inc, 2008; 509-520.

6. Wilczynski NL, Morgan D, Haynes RB; Hedges Team. An overview of the design and methods for retrieving high-quality studies for clinical care. *BMC Med Inform Decis Mak.* 2005;5:20.

7. Wilczynski NL, Haynes RB, Hedges Team. Developing optimal search strategies for detecting clinically sound prognostic studies in MEDLINE: an analytic survey. *BMC Med.* 2004;2:23.

8. Walker-Dilks C, Wilczynski NL, Haynes RB; Hedges Team. Cumulative Index to Nursing and Allied Health Literature search strategies for identifying methodologically sound causation and prognosis studies. *Appl Nurs Res.* 2008;21:98-103.

9. Wilczynski NL, Haynes RB. Optimal search strategies for detecting clinically sound prognostic studies in EMBASE: an analytic survey. *J Am Med Inform Assoc.* 2005;12:481-485.

6

Clinical Prediction Guides

Nancy Wilczynski

INTRODUCTION

When making a diagnosis or prognosis, or examining causes, or choosing treatment options, clinicians are often required to make predictions based on clinical history, physical examinations, and laboratory results. **Clinical prediction guides (CPGs)**, also known as clinical prediction rules or clinical decision rules, are increasingly sought by clinicians to assist in the decision making process.[1-3] The objective of CPGs is to reduce the uncertainty in clinical decision making by defining how to use clinical findings to make predictions. CPGs can help clinicians identify patients who require diagnostic tests, treatment, or hospitalization, and provide an objective standard by which to gauge which elements in a patient's history, physical examination, and laboratory tests are the most important in forming an accurate clinical assessment.[3]

CLINICAL EXAMPLE

Once again, as in previous chapters, we will start with an example of a problem and the research that went into solving it. Sciolla and colleagues[4] undertook a study to prospectively validate the ABCD score in a population of patients accessing emergency departments. The ABCD score is a 6-point score based on age, blood pressure, clinical features, and duration that previously had been shown to effectively stratify the short-term risk of stroke after transient ischemic attack (TIA). Validating the score was important, as clinicians could use this score to predict which patients were more likely to have a stroke and hence follow them more carefully. Those patients at lower risk could be reassured and resources needed for follow-up could be used where they are needed more. In addition to validating the ABCD score, Sciolla and colleagues set out to determine if adding computed tomography (CT) scan findings to the score would improve its performance. During a 6-month period, all TIA patients accessing the emergency departments in 13 hospitals in northern Italy were prospectively enrolled and stratified according to the 6-point ABCD score and to a 7-point score (ABCDI, where I = imaging) incorporating CT findings. Among the 274 enrolled patients, stroke occurred in 10 patients (3.6%) within 7 days and in 15 patients (5.5%) within 30 days. The authors found that the ABCD score was predictive of stroke at both 7 and 30 days and that including the CT scan findings increased prediction. The authors concluded that their study confirmed the prognostic value of the ABCD score in a prospective cohort of patients accessing emergency departments, and that incorporating CT results could further improve prediction.

HOW CLINICAL PREDICTION GUIDE STUDIES ARE DONE

CPGs are created and tested in 3 steps:

1. Deriving the guide or rule using current or future patients or data sets of previous patients
2. Testing or validating the rule (the validation process may require several studies in order to fully test the accuracy of the guide at different clinical sites)
3. Assessing the impact of the rule on clinical behavior (impact analysis)[3]

CPGs are derived from systematic clinical observations. CPG developers begin by constructing a list of potential predictors (e.g., age) of the outcome of interest (e.g., stroke).[3] The list typically includes items from the patient history and physical exam, and laboratory tests. The study investigators then examine a group of patients and determine if the potential predictors are present and the patient's status on the outcome of interest.[3] Statistical analysis reveals which factors are the most powerful predictors, and which factors can be omitted from the clinical prediction guide or rule without loss of predictive power.[4] Typically, the statistical techniques used in this process are based on logistic regression.

METHODOLOGICAL ISSUES

According to the *Users' Guides for CPGs*[3] there are 4 criteria that should be considered when assessing the methodologic standards for validation of a CPG:

- Were the patients chosen in an unbiased fashion and do they represent a wide spectrum of severity of disease?
- Was there a blinded assessment of the criterion standard for all patients?
- Was there an explicit and accurate interpretation of the predictor variables and the actual rule without knowledge of the outcome?
- Was there 100% follow up of those enrolled?

CPGs that have been derived but not tested or validated are often published but should not be considered ready for clinical application. Ideally, a validation of the rule entails the study investigators applying the guide prospectively in a new population (as in our clinical example) with a different prevalence and spectrum of disease from that of the patients in whom the guide was derived.[3] It is important to determine if the CPG performs similarly in a variety of populations, in the hands of a variety of clinicians, working in a variety of settings or institutions.[3]

AVAILABILITY OF CPGs

CPGs that are currently available cover a wide range of topics. For example, CPGs help to establish the pretest probability of pulmonary embolus,[5] to determine the treatment for pharyngitis,[6] and to rule out the need for unnecessary radiography for knee injuries ("Ottawa Knee Rule").[7] CPGs vary in complexity, but those that require simple calculations on the part of the user are most recommended by CPG advocates.[8]

A library of CPGs can be found at the Mount Sinai School of Medicine Evidence-based Medicine website (http://www.mssm.edu/medicine/general-medicine/ebm/#cpr). The CPGs listed were chosen by a team of academic general internists for common medical problems (e.g., probability of pneumonia, if an x-ray is needed for ankle pain). They are organized by level of evidence, a measure of quality that describes whether the CPG is merely derived (level 4) or validated (levels 2 to 3), or whether an impact analysis of the CPG has been done (i.e., assessing the impact of the rule on clinical behavior) (level 1).[5] CPGs can also be downloaded to PDA devices from this website.

SUMMARY

CPGs can serve as decision aids for determination of causation, diagnosis, prognosis, or patient responsiveness to treatment.[1-3] CPG advocates state that, when rigorously created and appropriately applied, CPGs have the potential to influence clinical opinion, change clinical behavior, and increase efficiency while preserving or improving quality patient care and satisfaction.[5]

SEARCHING METHODOLOGY

Now that we have summarized the components of clinical prediction guide studies, we move onto searching for CPGs in the large electronic databases such as MEDLINE. This task can be challenging but using search terms that target the methodology specific to CPG development in addition to content terms (e.g., stroke) can aid in retrieval effectiveness. The search terms available to use in 4 of the large electronic databases follow. The terms were compiled during the Clinical Hedges Study[9] after seeking input from clinicians and librarians in the United States and Canada. Index terms, subheadings, and publication types are assigned to each article in the database by staff working for the electronic database (e.g., MEDLINE). Textwords are used to search for articles using the article title and the article abstract. Preferred search terms are shown for MEDLINE and EMBASE, as search strategies were developed for detecting CPGs during the Clinical Hedges Study for these databases.

MEDLINE

MeSH, Subheadings, Publication Types, and Textwords

MeSH (Medical Subject Headings — Index Terms)

Observer variation*
Predictive value of tests*

Algorithms
Cohort studies (can be exploded)
Decision support techniques (can be exploded)
Decision trees
Follow-up studies
Forecasting
Guidelines
Logistic models
Longitudinal studies (can be exploded)
Probability (can be exploded)
Prospective studies
Reproducibility of results
Risk (can be exploded)
Risk assessment
Risk factors
"Sensitivity and specificity" (can be exploded)
Time factors

Subheadings

None

---

*Indicates a preferred term as determined in the Clinical Hedges Study.[10]

Publication Types

None

Textwords (Same List Is Used for All 4 Databases)

Develop*
Index*
Model*
Observ:*
Predict:*
Prediction*
Scor::*
Validat:*
Validation*
Validate*

Bootstrap technique
Boot-strap technique
Bootstrapping
Boot-strapping
Clinical criteri:
Clinical decision rule:
Clinical prediction index
Clinical prediction indices
Clinical prediction instrument:
Clinical prediction model:
Clinical prediction rule:
Clinical prediction tool:
Clinical predictor:
Clinical predictor variable:
Clinical score:
Clinical tool:
Cohort:
Cohort stud:
Create rule:
Created rule:
Creating rule:
Decision rule:
Derivat:
Derivation cohort:
Derivation sample:
Derivation set:

Derive rule
Derived rule
Deriving rule
Discriminant analys:
Equation:
Formula:
Guide:
Impact analysis
Index
Indices
Likelihood ratio:
Logistic
Logistic analys:
Logistic regression
Logistic:
Model:
Multivariate logistic analys:
Neural network:
Outcome predict:
Outcome stud:
Prediction guide:
Prediction index
Prediction indices
Prediction instrument:
Prediction model:
Prediction rule:
Prediction tool:
Predictive
Predictive guide:
Predictive instrument:
Predictive model:
Predictive power
Predictive rule:
Predictive value
Predictor:
Predictor variable:
ROC
Receiver operating curve:
Receiver operator curve:
Recursive partitioning analys:
Relative risk
RR
Risk
Rule:

Rule assessment
Rule assessment tool:
Scoring system
Sensitivity
Specificity
Test:
Test rule:
Tested rule:
Testing rule:
Test set:
Testing set:
Training:
Training cohort:
Training sample:
Training set:
Validated criteri:
Validate rule:
Validated rule:
Validating rule:
Validat: rule
Validation cohort:
Validation phase:
Validation sample:
Validation set:

CINAHL (CUMULATIVE INDEX TO NURSING AND ALLIED HEALTH LITERATURE)

Index Terms, Subheadings, and Publication Types

Index Terms

Algorithms
Apgar score
Clinical assessment tools (can be exploded)
Decision making, clinical
Discriminant analysis
Forecasting
Independent variable
Instrument validation
Logistic regression (can be exploded)
Multivariate analysis
"Neural networks (computer)"

"Outcomes (health care)" (can be exploded)
Outcomes research
Predictive value of tests
Probability
Prospective studies (can be exploded)
Relative risk
Reproducibility of results
Risk assessment
Risk factors (can be exploded)
"Rules and regulations"
"Sensitivity and specificity"
Time factors

Subheadings

None

Publication Types

None

EMBASE

Index Terms, Subheadings, and Publication Types

Index Terms

Methodology (can be exploded)*

Algorithm
Apgar score
Artificial neural network
Cell specificity
Chronology
Clinical feature
Clinical practice
Clinical study (can be exploded)
Cohort analysis
Computer analysis
Cosmological phenomena (can be exploded)

---

*Indicates a preferred term as determined in the Clinical Hedges Study.[11]

Decision making
Decision theory
Diagnostic accuracy
Diagnostic test (can be exploded)
Discriminant analysis
Drug specificity
Epidemiology (can be exploded)
Follow up
Forecasting
Futurology (can be exploded)
Heart index
Incubation time
Labeling index
Long term care (can be exploded)
Longitudinal study
Mathematical phenomena (can be exploded)
Medical decision making
Model (can be exploded)
Multivariate analysis (can be exploded)
Nerve cell network
Practice guideline (can be exploded)
Prediction and forecasting
Prediction
Probability
Prospective study
Receiver operating characteristic
Regression analysis
Reproducibililty
Risk assessment
Risk factor
Risk (can be exploded)
Scoring system
Sensitivity and sensibility
Statistical analysis (can be exploded)
Statistical concepts (can be exploded)
Statistical model
Statistical parameters (can be exploded)
Symptomatology (can be exploded)
Time
Training
Treatment outcome (can be exploded)
Unclassified drug
Validation process

Subheadings

None

Publication Types

None

PsycINFO

Index Terms, Subheadings, and Publication Types

Index Terms

Algorithms
Cohort analysis
Decision support systems
Followup studies
Item analysis, statistical
Item response theory
Longitudinal studies (can be exploded)
Mathematical modeling (can be exploded)
Maximum likelihood
Multiple regression
Multivariate analysis (can be exploded)
Neural networks
Predictability, measurement
Prediction (can be exploded)
Prediction errors (can be exploded)
Probability (can be exploded)
Prospective studies
Risk analysis
Risk factors
Statistical analysis(can be exploded)
Statistical estimation (can be exploded)
Statistical regression (can be exploded)
Statistical validity
Structural equation modeling
Treatment effectiveness evaluation
Treatment guidelines

Subheadings

None

Publication Types

Followup study
Longitudinal study

EXAMPLES OF TEXTWORDS AND INDEXING USING OUR CLINICAL EXAMPLE

Citation for Our Clinical Example

Sciolla R, Melis F; SINPAC Group. Rapid identification of high-risk transient ischemic attacks: prospective validation of the ABCD score. *Stroke.* 2008;39:297–302.

Textwords and Index Terms Used in Our Clinical Example

Textwords (in the Title and Abstract of the Article)

Predict:*
Prediction*
Scor::*
Validat:*
Validate*
Validation*

Cohort:
Predictive
Risk

MEDLINE INDEXING

Predictive value of tests*

Follow-up studies
Prospective studies
Risk factors

CINAHL INDEXING

Predictive value of tests
Prospective studies
Risk factors

---

*Indicates a preferred term as determined in the Clinical Hedges Study[10,11]

PROVEN STRATEGIES

Search Strategies (Filters) Derived during the Clinical Hedges Study [10,11]

Filter*	MEDLINE (Ovid syntax)	EMBASE (Ovid syntax)
Sensitive	predict:.mp. OR scor:.tw. OR observ:mp.	predict:.tw. OR exp methodology OR validat:.tw.
Specific	validation.tw. OR validate.tw.	validation.tw. OR prediction.tw.
Minimize difference between Sensitivity and Specificity	predict:tw. OR validat:.mp. OR develop.tw.	validat:.mp. OR index.tw. OR model.tw.

*See the Introduction for a description of how to use these filters and where to find them in Ovid and PubMed.

LINKS TO OTHER RESOURCES

Link to information regarding the Clinical Hedges Study: http://hiru.mcmaster.ca/hiru/HIRU_Hedges_home.aspx

Link to how to use an article about CPGs: http://www.cche.net/usersguides/prediction.asp

EXERCISES

Note that the search possibilities (answers) are detailed in the Appendix.

1. Is there a tool for predicting the probability of sentinel lymph node metastasis in breast cancer?
2. Is there a tool to predict functional decline in older adults who have been discharged from the emergency department?

REFERENCES

1. Laupacis A, Sekar N, Stiell IG. Clinical prediction rules. A review and suggested modifications of methodological standards. *JAMA*. 1997;277:488–494.
2. Wasson JH, Sox HC, Neff RK, Goldman L. Clinical prediction rules. Applications and methodological standards. *N Engl J Med*. 1985;313:793–799.
3. Guyatt G, Rennie D, Meade MO, Cook DJ. *Users' Guide to the Medical Literature. A Manual for Evidence-Based Clinical Practice*. 2 ed. New York, NY: McGraw-Hill Companies Inc, 2008; 491–505.

4. Sciolla R, Melis F; SINPAC Group. Rapid identification of high-risk transient ischemic attacks: prospective validation of the ABCD score. *Stroke.* 2008;39:297–302.

5. Wells PS, Ginsberg JS, Anderson DR, et al. Use of a clinical model for safe management of patients with suspected pulmonary embolism. *Ann Intern Med.* 1998;129:997–1005.

6. Walsh BT, Bookheim WW, Johnson RC, Tompkins RK. Recognition of streptococcal pharyngitis in adults. *Arch Intern Med.* 1975;135:1493–1497.

7. Emparanza JI, Aginaga JR, Estudio Multicentro en Urgencias de Osakidetza: Reglas de Ottawa (EMUORO) Group. Validation of the Ottawa Knee Rules. *Ann Emerg Med.* 2001;38:364–368.

8. McGinn T. Practice corner: using clinical prediction rules. *ACP J Club.* 2002;137:A11–12.

9. Wilczynski NL, Morgan D, Haynes RB; Hedges Team. An overview of the design and methods for retrieving high-quality studies for clinical care. *BMC Med Inform Decis Mak.* 2005;5:20.

10. Wong SS, Wilczynski NL, Haynes RB, Ramkissoonsingh R; Hedges Team. Developing optimal search strategies for detecting sound clinical prediction studies in MEDLINE. *AMIA Annu Symp Proc.* 2003:728–732.

11. Holland JL, Wilczynski NL, Haynes RB; Hedges Team. Optimal search strategies for identifying sound clinical prediction studies in EMBASE. *BMC Med Inform Decis Mak.* 2005;5:11.

7

Decision Analyses

Ann McKibbon

INTRODUCTION

Decision making in modern health care is becoming more complex. At the same time, individual patients and their families are taking, or being given, more responsibility in making decisions concerning their health and well being. Both clinicians and patients have traditional information resources to help them sort out the risks and benefits of the available options or choices. Many options now exist in health care as we know it. For example, decisions concerning breast cancer treatment include options of no treatment, minimal surgery, radical surgery, chemotherapy, radiation therapy, or combinations of several of these treatments. In addition, the combinations can involve different timing choices and the sequence the steps can take.

Two advances that can help in clinical decision making are **patient decision aids** and formal **decision analyses**. Patient decision aids are tools that present the available options to the patient and his or her caregivers. The potential options include the risks and benefits for each option and some idea of how common these risks (e.g., death or disability) and benefits (e.g., disease-free survival or cure) will likely be (i.e., how probable are they likely to occur). A well-designed patient decision aid will also allow the patient to consider how important each of the benefits and risks are to her or him and factor these into the decision. Patient decision aids are meant to supplement and enhance interaction with health professionals and not replace the clinicians during the decision-making process. The Ottawa Health Research Institute has done considerable work in collecting and assessing patient decision aids. Their website[1] provides a valuable resource for anyone interested in the decision aids themselves or in their development and evaluation.

Formal decision analyses take these patient decision aids one step further. They map out or model the decisions and place formal values on the benefits and harms, much like some of the major patient decision aids. The formal decision analyses allow calculation of preferred options based on patient and provider preferences. They allow quantification of benefits and projections of the costs and outcomes, and incorporate the importance each of these outcomes. Formal decision analyses are used in a wider range of situations than patient decision aids. They are also widely used in other domains such as business, manufacturing, and engineering. The remainder of the chapter will concentrate on formal decision analyses, although the clinical example studies both patient decision aids and formal decision analyses. Again, for those interested in patient decision aids refer to the Ottawa Health Research Institute web site (http://decisionaid.ohri.ca/).

CLINICAL EXAMPLE

Mothers who have had a caesarean section for the birth of their first child need to make decisions about the mode of delivery of subsequent babies. In the past "once a caesarean, always a caesarean" was the usual wisdom. This is now no longer the case and many women successfully have a vaginal delivery after emergency sections. Caesarean sections, either planned or emergency, hold more risks to the mother and infant and consume more health care resources than standard vaginal deliveries. Planning the optimal mode of delivery requires careful consideration by both the mother and her partner. The final decision of the planned delivery mode must account for family and individual preferences. In addition to the family's preferences, the health providers can add clinical information on the woman's existing conditions that increase the risk of a second caesarean section. Montgomery and colleagues [2] wanted to determine how best to provide planning information to pregnant women and their partners for sorting out delivery choices.

Using strong methods of randomized controlled trials, the study investigators sought to determine if 2 potential information methods were more effective at reducing decisional conflict in the mothers, and if the methods led to different proportions of planned vaginal births, planned caesarean sections, and emergency caesarean sections. The first method of imparting information to women was a patient decision aid that provided information on options (planned delivery modes) and their benefits and risks. In addition to the benefits and risks, the probabilities of having outcomes and their severity were also given. These outcomes included such things as pain and need for pain medication, length of hospital stay, and infections related to surgery for vaginal delivery vs planned and emergency sections.

The second method of providing information was a formal decision analysis. This decision analysis showed the women and their partners the options, the outcomes and their probabilities, and factored in the values that the individual woman or couple placed on various outcomes and benefits. A "decision tree" was drawn and a simple computer analysis provided a numerical weighting of the best path or set of options based on how the woman valued each of the factors in the decision. The woman could modify her values and a new "best path" was presented. The woman continued until she was comfortable with her decision making in relation to mode of delivery.

These 2 information-sharing methods were compared with usual care by midwives and physicians. Consecutive women were recruited during a clinic visit when they were 10 to 20 weeks pregnant. Of the 1148 women who were invited to be in the study, 742 women agreed and were randomized to 1 of the 3 groups: usual care, patient decision aid, or formal decision analysis. The decision aid and decision analysis program were available online. No mode of delivery was advocated for any of the 3 groups—the woman made her own decision regarding plans for the delivery. The midwives and physicians responsible for their care helped implement the women's choices. Just before delivery (around 37 weeks of gestation), the women filled in questionnaires regarding their decisional conflict over the delivery decision. The details of the delivery were collected after birth.

Both the decision aid and decision analysis were associated with greater knowledge and less anxiety and decisional conflict concerning the delivery compared with usual care. Slightly more women in the decision analysis group had vaginal deliveries. Although the researchers showed that both the patient decision aid and the formal decision analysis were better than usual care for lessening decisional conflict, the findings of the study could not determine if the decision aid or decision analysis was better or preferred.

METHODOLOGICAL ISSUES

The clinical example shows some of the important features of a formal decision analysis:

- Various options or choices exist and one is not necessarily better than another.
- People perceive outcomes and risks differently. How an individual values things like potential for pain, increased hospital stays, likelihood of surgery or radiation can be factored into the decision-making process.
- The options, outcomes, potential for benefits and risks, and values can be given weights. All of these can be analyzed taking into account costs (dollars, time, and use of resources), and a preferred route or option sequence can be calculated for each patient. To say it another way, the decision that a patient needs to make entails tradeoffs between options that have varying advantages and disadvantages.

HISTORY OF DECISION ANALYSES

Because of the work done on code breaking during World War II, the discipline of information sciences blossomed and grew in scope and importance in the 1940s and 1950s. Two branches of information sciences developed in the 1950s: game theory and decision theory. Decision analyses have their foundation in these areas of study as well as philosophy, and their domains formalized the methods and approaches of decision analyses. Formal decision analyses are heavily used in business and manufacturing. An industrial example of an application of an industrial decision analysis would be a computer program that provided data that suggested which type of automobile would be best made at each plant of an automotive company and if a third shift is justified above the usual 2 shifts of production workers. It was not until the late 1960s that health care, especially medicine, started to use decision analyses.

Mainframe computer use grew in the 1980s and some early decision analyses were developed and implemented. Because relatively few computers existed and their speed and power were limited, these early decision analyses were often quite simplistic. Another surge in decision analyses occurred in the 1990s with the advent of the personal computers. Decision analyses became more common and complex in health care. The early years of the 21st century saw many implementations of powerful electronic health records. Again the development and use of decision analyses surged as they became embedded into the electronic health records and were harnessed to direct individual patient decision making.

STEPS IN DEVELOPING A FORMAL DECISION ANALYSIS

Detsky and colleagues[3-7] have written a series of journal articles on medical decision analyses. These articles describe decision analyses for those who are interested in producing their own analyses, as well as provide valuable information for those who simply want to understand how decision analyses work. The first step in the production of a decision analysis is to choose the clinical situation and describe the choices. The next step is to build a decision tree.

A decision tree is built using symbols, lines, and numbers. The lines are strategy or decision paths. The lines branch out and often represent the options available for consideration. The paths are built using choice nodes (symbolized by squares), chance nodes (symbolized by circles), and outcomes (symbolized by triangles). Numbers associated with lines are probabilities of the outcomes. Numbers associated with triangles (outcomes) are the numbers that are associated with the "utilities" or values placed on outcomes, both good and bad, by the person making the decision. Utilities have a number ranging from 1, which is often defined as perfect health, to 0, which is often defined as death. A small number of decision trees have used negative utilities indicating a situation that a patient describes as worse than death.

To show how a very simple tree diagram is drawn, the following hypothetical information is available.

A patient has a choice of surgery or chemotherapy for her cancer:

- Surgery is associated with
  - 2% chance of dying from the operation (life expectancy 0 years)
  - 50% chance of being cured (life expectancy 15 years)
  - 48% chance of not being cured (life expectancy 1 year)
- Chemotherapy is associated with
  - 5% chance of death (life expectancy 0 years)
  - 65% chance of cure (life expectancy 15 years)
  - 30% chance of having the cancer progression slowed (life expectancy 2 years)

Note that for each choice the probability of the outcomes must add up to 1.00. That means that each option or branching of the decision analysis tree must include all of the outcomes that are possible (Figure 7-1A and B).

- The 2 options are surgery or chemotherapy (squares)
- The chance notes (circles) are given for each option
- The outcomes are death, cure, not being cured, and slowed progression of the cancer (triangles)

Calculation using the time gained in Figure 7-1A is done by taking each arm (surgery and chemotherapy) and summing the product of the probability and the time gained. This calculation provides the average life gains for each option.

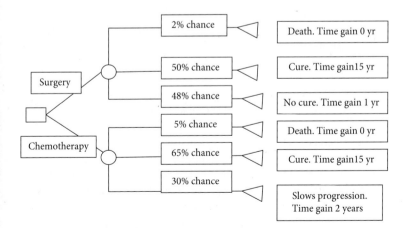

Figure 7-1A. Decision tree for hypothetical decision of surgery or chemotherapy for cancer showing time gained with each option and outcome.

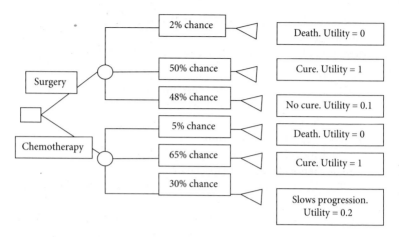

Figure 7-1B. Decision tree for hypothetical decision of surgery or chemotherapy for cancer showing the utility of each outcome (one person's value of each outcome).

For the surgery option the calculation with respect to time gained is:
(Probability of death × 0 year) + (Probability of cure × 15 year) + (Probability of no cure × 1 year)
= (0.02 × 0) + (0.5 × 15) + (0.48 × 1)
= 0 + 7.5 + 0.48
= 7.98 or almost 8 years gained on average with a choice of surgery for the cancer compared with no surgery or chemotherapy

For the chemotherapy option the calculation on time gained is:
(Probability of death × 0 year) + (Probability of cure × 15 years) + (Probability of slowed disease progression × 2 years)
= (0.05 × 0) + (0.65 × 15) + (0.30 × 2)
= 0 + 9.75 + 0.6
= 10.35 years gained on average for a choice of chemotherapy for the cancer compared with no surgery of chemotherapy

The difference between these 2 calculations (10.35 – 7.98) show that on average a person will gain 2.37 years of life by selecting the chemotherapy option. This method of calculation does not take into account how the person involved values each of the outcomes. Usually the value is 1 for perfect health and 0 for death. In our example (Figure7-1B) the person making the surgery vs chemotherapy decision uses the standard values for death and cure. She also puts a value of 0.1 on no cure and 0.2 on slowed progression. Once again we do the calculation using the values or utilities instead of time summing the products of the 3 outcomes time utilities for each option.

For the surgery option the calculation using utilities is:
(Probability of death × Utility of death) + (Probability of cure × Utility of cure) + (Probability of no cure × Utility of no cure)

= (0.02 × 0) + (0.5 × 1) + (0.48 × 0.1)

= 0 + 0.5 + 0.048

= 0.55 (rounded up to 2 decimal places)

For the chemotherapy option the calculation for utilities is
(Probability of death × Utility of death) + (Probability of cure × Utility of cure) + (Probability of slowed progression × Utility of slowed progression)

= (0.05 × 0) + (0.65 × 1) + (0.30 × 0. 2)

= 0 + .65 + 0.06

= 0.71

The chemotherapy option has substantially more utility than the surgery option.

In this example the person should seriously consider the chemotherapy option as it provides both an average life savings of over 2 years and a fairly substantial increase in the utility of chemotherapy. Many decision trees are much more complicated, with multiple options and outcomes. Because of their branching nature and the use of numbers and probabilities, one can see how well tree diagrams in formal decision analyses are suited for computerization.

Once decision tress become too complex researchers often build computer models of the decision-making process. These can be Markov models, neural networks, or influence diagrams. These are beyond the scope of this book but the terms are listed so that you will know that they are more advanced topics of formal decision analyses. As an example of decision-making complexities, Figure 7-2 shows an influence diagram to determine resource allocation for AIDS programs in southern Africa.[8]

Formal decision analyses, like patient decision aids, can be used with individual patients and families to make a decision in relation to a disease or condition. Formal decision analyses are also useful for classes of problems, such as the choice of hormone replacement after the results of the Women's Health Initiative trials were released.[9] Decision analyses can also help decide policy, such as early hospital discharge after uncomplicated myocardial infarction[10] or vaccination for Lyme disease.[11] Although they are often used in treatment decisions, decision analyses can also be applied to diagnostic and other decisions. For example, in the case of determining the best approach to diagnose patients with unexpected weight loss, a decision analysis showed that a 2-step approach was most cost effective.[12] Decision analyses can also affect national decisions such as mammography or colorectal cancer screening. The following health care areas have harnessed formal decision analyses well. Some of the domains are important

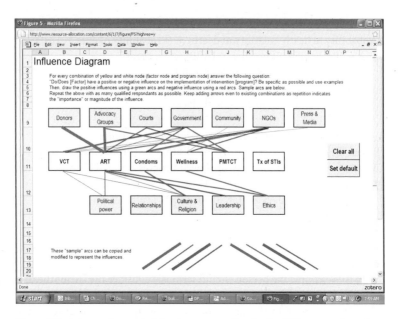

Figure 7-2. Influence diagram to determine resource allocation for AIDS programs in southern Africa.[8]

to decision making for populations and policies. Others are important for individual patient decision making.

- Economic analyses of all kinds—especially when intending to combine costs and outcomes in one analysis
- Health technology assessments
- Treatment
  - ○ Choosing between treatments including no-treatment options
  - ○ Sequencing of therapies

- Prevention
  - ○ Showing an individual what happens if they incorporate weight loss, exercise, or diet modifications

- Showing progression of disease and probable/possible outcomes
- Diagnosis
  - ○ Sequencing of tests
  - ○ Defining the context in which a test is useful
  - ○ Choosing among tests including no-test options
  - ○ Testing to guide treatments, for example, measuring blood coagulation times in the use of warfarin for patients with atrial fibrillation
- Screening decisions for populations

SUMMARY

Formal decision analyses are processes that can be used to estimate overall expected benefits and harms, or to compare the costs and benefits of complex alternative choices in the health care of individuals and populations. They are related to patient decision aids but are often more complex and with a broader range of applications. Many domains such as manufacturing and engineering use decision analysis techniques. Once a decision situation is identified that has acceptable options, a decision tree or other model is produced. Various values (utilities) can be entered into the system and alternatives analyzed. With the increasing number of electronic health record systems and the power of the Internet, formal decision analyses will only grow in importance.

SEARCHING METHODOLOGY

No proven strategies exist for formal decision analyses. Searching Can be difficult for this material. In addition no subheadings, publication types, or other searching methods are useful beyond index terms and textwords. Also use terms given in the chapter on economics (Chapter 12) and health technology assessments (Chapter 13).

Textwords (Same List Is Used for All 4 Databases)

Decision analys:
Decision making
Model:
Bayes theorem
Markov model:
Decision analytic model:
Decision model:
Decision tree:
Influence diagram:

MEDLINE TERMS

Bayes theorem
Data interpretation, statistical
Decision making (can be exploded)
Decision support systems, clinical
Decision support systems, management
Decision support techniques (can be exploded)
Decision theory
Decision trees

Game theory (can be exploded)
Models, biologic
Models, economic
Models, organizational
Models, statistical (can be exploded)
Neural networks (computer)
Risk
Risk assessment

CINAHL TERMS

Decision making (can be exploded)
Decision making, clinical
Decision making, computer assisted
Decision support techniques (can be exploded)
Decision support techniques, clinical
Decision support techniques, management
Decision trees
Models theoretical
Models, statistical
Neural networks, computer

EMBASE TERMS

Decision support system
Decision theory
Theoretical model
Decision making
Risk management
Bayes theorem
Artificial neural network
Hidden markov model
Computer model
Mathematical computing

PsycINFO TERMS

Decision support systems
Decision theory
Decision making
Information processing model
Markov chains
Mathematical models
Game theory

EXAMPLES OF TEXTWORDS AND INDEXING USING OUR CLINICAL EXAMPLE

Citation for Our Clinical Example 1

Ghori AK, Chung KC. A decision-analysis model to diagnose feigned hand weakness. J Hand Surg—American volume. 32(10):1638-1643.

Textwords and Index Terms Used in Our Clinical Example
Textwords (in the Title and Abstract of the Article)

Decision analysis
Model

MEDLINE INDEXING

Decision support techniques

EMBASE INDEXING

Decision making

Citation for Our Clinical Example 2

Borsuk M, Mauer M, Leinert J. Larsen TA. Charting a path for innovative toilet technology using multicriteria decision analyses. Environ Sci Technol. 2008;42(6):1855-1862.

Textwords and Index Terms Used in Our Clinical Example
Textwords (in the Title and Abstract of the Article)

Decision analysis
Multicriteria decision analysis
Alternative

MEDLINE INDEXING

Decision support techniques

EMBASE INDEXING

Decision making
Risk management

Citation for Our Clinical Example 3

Chang K-Y, Chan K-H, Chang S-H, Yang M-C, Chen TH-H. Decision analysis for epidural labor analgesia with Multiattribute Utility (MAU) Model. Clin J Pain. 2008;24(3):265-272.

Textwords and Index Terms Used in Our Clinical Example

Textwords (in the Title and Abstract of the Article)

Decision analysis
Multiattribute utility

MEDLINE INDEXING

Decision support techniques
Models, biologic

CINAHL INDEXING

Decision making
Utility theory

EMBASE INDEXING

Decision making
Theoretical model

PROVEN STRATEGIES

We are not aware of published search filters. Jerome[13] has produced a brief introduction to searching for decision analyses; however, it concentrates on economic analyses. Decision analyses are broader in scope although economics is an important component.

LINK TO OTHER RESOURCES

Ottawa Health Research Institute, Patient Decision Aids web site: http://decisionaid.ohri.ca/

EXERCISES

Note that the search possibilities (answers) are detailed in the Appendix.

1. For geriatric patients what diseases and conditions have been studied using formal decision analyses?
2. What do formal decision analyses say about treating otitis media in children with respect to antibiotics, tubes, and no treatment?

REFERENCES

1. Ottawa Health Research Institute. Patient Decision Aids. http://decisionaid. ohri.ca/. Accessed September 13. 2008.

2. Montgomery AA, Emmett CL, Fahey T, Jones C, Ricketts I, Patel RR, Peters TJ, Murphy DJ, on behalf of the DIAMOND Study Group. Two decision aids for mode of delivery among women with previous caesarean section: randomised controlled trial. *BMJ*. 2007;334:1305-1312.

3. Detsky AS, Naglie G, Krahn MD, Naimark D, Redelmeier DA. Primer on medical decision analysis: Part 1—Getting started. *Med Decis Making*. 1997;17:123-125.

4. Detsky AS, Naglie G, Krahn MD, Redelmeier DA, Naimark D. Primer on medical decision analysis: Part 2—Building a tree. *Med Decis Making*. 1997;17:126-135.

5. Naglie G, Krahn MD, Naimark D, Redelmeier DA, Detsky AS. Primer on medical decision analysis: Part 3—Estimating probabilities and utilities. *Med Decis Making*. 1997;17:136-141.

6. Krahn MD, Naglie G, Naimark D, Redelmeier DA, Detsky AS. Primer on medical decision analysis: Part 4—Analyzing the model and interpreting the results. *Med Decis Making*. 1997;17:142-151.

7. Naimark D, Krahn MD, Naglie G, Redelmeier DA, Detsky AS. Primer on medical decision analysis: Part 5—Working with Markov processes. *Med Decis Making*. 1997;17:152-159.

8. Lasry A, Carter MW, Zaric GS. S4HARA: System for HIV/AIDS resource allocation. *Cost Eff Resource Alloc*. 2008;6:7.

9. Newby LK, Eisenstein EL, Califf RM, et al. Cost effectiveness of early discharge after uncomplicated acute myocardial infarction. *N Engl J Med*. 2000;342:749-755.

10. Hsia EC, Chung JB, Schwartz JS, Albert DA. Cost-effectiveness analysis of the Lyme disease vaccine. *Arthritis Rheum*. 2002;46:1439-1442.

11. Lankisch P, Gerzmann M, Gerzmann JF, Lehnick D. Unintentional weight loss: diagnosis and prognosis. The first prospective follow up study from a secondary referral centre. *J Inter Med*. 2001;249:41-46.

12. Kim C, Kwok YS. Decision analysis of hormone replacement therapy after Women's Health Initiative. *Am J Obstet Gynecol*. 2003;189:1228-1233.

13. Jerome RB. Decision analysis: A brief introduction for the searcher. *MLA News*. 2008;Apr(405):14-15.

8

Differential Diagnosis and Disease Manifestation

Nancy Wilczynski

INTRODUCTION

Differential diagnosis involves the process of weighing the probability that 1 disease rather than another disease accounts for a patient's illness. During the process of arriving at a final diagnosis, the clinician observes the patient's signs and symptoms, considers the most likely illnesses, and then narrows down the possible diagnoses. For example, when presented with a patient with rhinitis (a runny nose), the clinician would consider allergic rhinitis (hay fever), the abuse of nasal decongestants, and the common cold as likely illnesses. The clinician needs to distinguish among the diseases that have similar characteristics by comparing and contrasting their signs and symptoms. In order to classify the patient's signs and symptoms into a disease, the clinician needs to know the **clinical manifestations of each disease** that he/she is expected to diagnose. The terms *clinical manifestations* and *clinical findings* are generally used interchangeably and refer to findings the clinician can gather directly from the patient, usually during the medical interview or physical examination. These clinical findings can be further divided into those that the patient reports (symptoms) and those that the clinician ascertains by using skills or equipment such as a stethoscope (signs).

Another way of understanding the difference between diagnosis and differential diagnosis is that diagnosis studies take patients with a set of signs and symptoms and tries to sort out what single disease is causing the problems. Differential diagnosis using disease manifestation knowledge and other aspects of the patients and their conditions takes patients with a single main complaint such as children with fever of unknown origin, syncope (fainting), unintentional weight loss or gain, and quite often certain aspects of pain or discomfort. The differential diagnosis study tries to sort out what proportion of the patients with the single sign or symptom has various diseases.

Disease manifestation studies try to sort out the frequency of the symptoms associated with a particular disease or condition. Disease manifestation data often are presented in table format. For example, Burbige and colleagues[1] determined that children with Crohn disease had the following characteristics.

- 86% had abdominal pain
- 83% had fever
- 72% had diarrhea
- 30% had growth retardation
- 25% had joint involvement
- 24% had anorectal disease
- 14% had bleeding
- 10% had rash, erythemia, or nodosum

CLINICAL EXAMPLE

As with other chapters, we begin with a clinical example, in this case, for differential diagnosis. The problem was that rheumatoid arthritis (RA) needs to be diagnosed early so that appropriate treatment can commence promptly as this leads to improved clinical outcomes. Conventional clinical examination and radiography had been shown to be not as sensitive as magnetic resonance imaging (MRI) for detecting inflammatory and destructive joint changes in RA. Duer and colleagues[2] undertook a study to investigate the value of MRI and whole body bone scintigraphy in the differential diagnosis of patients with unclassified arthritis. Patients with different types of arthritis need different treatments.

Forty-one patients with unclassified arthritis participated. MRI and whole body bone scintigraphy were performed. Two rheumatologists agreed on the most likely diagnosis and the patients were treated accordingly. A final diagnosis was made by a specialist 2 years later. Tentative diagnoses after MRI and bone scintigraphy were: 13 patients with RA, 8 with osteoarthritis, 11 with other inflammatory diseases, and 9 with arthralgias without inflammatory or degenerative origin. Two years later, 11 of 13 patients originally assigned the tentative diagnosis of RA fulfilled the American College of Rheumatology (ACR) criteria, while 2 patients were reclassified. No patients given the non-RA diagnosis fulfilled the ACR criteria for RA at 2 years. The presence of MRI synovitis, MRI erosion, and bone scintigraphic pattern compatible with RA showed 100% specificity for a diagnosis of RA at 2 years follow-up. The authors concluded that MRI and bone scintigraphy findings were valuable in the differential diagnosis of patients with unclassified arthritis in routine clinical practice.

METHODOLOGY

User's guides for how to use disease probability for differential diagnosis and the clinical manifestations of disease are available through the Users' Guides Series to Evidence-Based Clinical Practice.[3] The guides highlight aspects of the study design that should be considered when determining the clinical applicability of an article. For example, when reviewing an article on using disease probability for differential diagnosis, the authors should explicitly state the criteria that were used for the final diagnosis. These criteria should include not only the findings needed to confirm each diagnosis, but also those findings useful for rejecting each diagnosis.[3] The *ACP Journal Club* also includes articles about differential diagnosis (http://www.acpjc.org/). The criteria used to determine eligibility for inclusion in the *ACP Journal Club* (i.e., determining if an article on differential diagnosis is methodologically rigorous) include:

- A cohort of patients who present with a similar, initially undiagnosed but reproducibly defined clinical problem
- An explicitly described clinical setting, including the referral filter (i.e., how were the patients identified and included into the study?)
- Ascertainment of diagnosis of ≥80% of patients using a reproducible diagnostic workup strategy for all patients, and follow-up until patients are diagnosed or, to minimize missed diagnoses, follow-up of ≥1 month for acute disorders or ≥1 year for chronic or relapsing disorders

Our clinical example meets all of these criteria.

Well-done studies of differential diagnosis reduce bias by having a prospective design, explicit diagnostic criteria, and standardized evaluations that are applied to a sufficient number of patients.[4] High-quality evidence about differential diagnosis can aid the clinician in making a final diagnosis because the probabilities of the disorders that cause the patient's presenting symptom or symptoms are reported. The number and percentages of patients who are found to have each underlying disorder are usually presented in the main results. These data can be used to estimate the disease probability of the disorder of interest for any 1 patient. Clinicians can use the disease probabilities as a starting point for estimating pretest probability in their own patients. Once the pretest probabilities have been estimated, they can be used to help with diagnostic decisions by assisting the clinician in deciding whether to pursue specific disorders as explanations for the patient's illness, choosing which diagnostic tests to order and how to interpret their results, and deciding whether to forego any testing and proceed with treatment.[4] See Chapter 3 to review how these pretest probabilities are used with likelihood ratios to help determine the post-test probability of whether the patient has or does not have the disease under investigation.

The users' guide for how to use an article on the clinical manifestations of disease[3] outlines how knowledge of the clinical manifestations of disease can be used in clinical diagnosis. This knowledge is useful when selecting a patient-specific differential diagnosis, when deciding whether to use further diagnostic testing, and when verifying a patient's final diagnosis. Additionally, knowledge of the clinical manifestations of disease is useful when initially evaluating the patient, as single findings and clusters of findings generate hypotheses of possible diagnoses.

The guide for how to use an article on the clinical manifestations of disease[3] also highlights aspects of the study design that should be considered when determining the clinical applicability of an article. For example, when evaluating the study sample, ideally the sample should mirror the whole population of those with the disease, so that the frequency of clinical manifestations in the sample approximates that of the population.[3] For a thorough overview, refer to the users' guide.[3]

SUMMARY

Differential diagnosis involves the process of weighing the probability that 1 disease rather than another disease accounts for a patient's illness, especially if 1 of the major signs or symptoms can be attributed to several diseases or conditions. The clinician needs to distinguish among the diseases that have similar characteristics by comparing and contrasting their signs and symptoms. In order to classify the patient's signs and symptoms into a disease, the clinician needs to know the clinical manifestations of each disease that he/she is expected to diagnose. Clinical manifestations of a disease refer to findings the clinicians can gather directly from the patient, usually during the medical interview or physical examination.

SEARCHING METHODOLOGY

Now that we have summarized the components of studies of differential diagnosis and disease manifestation, we move onto searching for these types of studies in the large electronic databases such as MEDLINE. This task can be challenging but using search terms that target the methodology specific to these types of studies in addition to your content terms (e.g., rheumatoid arthritis) can aid in retrieval effectiveness. The search terms available to use in 4 of the large electronic databases follow. The terms were compiled during the Clinical Hedges Study[7] after seeking input from clinicians and librarians in the United States and Canada. Index terms, subheadings, and publication types are assigned to each article in the database by staff working for the electronic database (e.g., MEDLINE). Textwords are used to search for articles using the article title and the article abstract. We are unable to show preferred search terms because search strategies derived to detect these types of studies were not developed during the Clinical Hedges Study. We present below possible terms based on the broad area of diagnosis.

MEDLINE

MeSH, Subheadings, Publication Types, and Textwords

MeSH (Medical Subject Headings — Index Terms)

Area under curve
Bayes theorem
Diagnosis (can be exploded)
Diagnosis, computer assisted (can be exploded)
Diagnosis, differential
Diagnosis, dual (psychiatry)
Diagnostic errors (can be exploded)
Diagnostic techniques and procedures (can be exploded)
False negative reactions
False positive reactions
Genetic testing
Laboratory techniques and procedures (can be exploded)
Likelihood functions
Mandatory testing
Mass chest x-ray
Mass screening (can be exploded)
Multiphasic screening
Neonatal screening
Observer variation
Odds ratio
Predictive value of tests
Probability (can be exploded)
Reference standards
ROC curve
Sensitivity and specificity (can be exploded)
Substance abuse detection
Vision screening

Subheadings

Diagnosis (for diagnosis of diseases and disorders) (can be exploded)
Diagnostic use (for substances used in diagnosis)

Publication Types

None

Textwords (Same List Is Used for All 4 Databases)

Area under the curve:
Accurac: (combination of sensitivity and specificity)
Accuracy
Clinical manifestation:
Criterion standard:
Diagnos:
Diagnostic standard:
Differential diagnosis
Disease manifestation:
False negative
False positive
False rate:
Gold standard:
Likelihood ratio:
Post test likelihood
Posttest likelihood
Post test probability
Posttest probability
Pre test likelihood
Predictive value:
Pretest likelihood
Receiver operat: curve:
ROC
Sensitiv:
Specificit:

CINAHL (CUMULATIVE INDEX TO NURSING AND ALLIED HEALTH LITERATURE)

Index Terms, Subheadings, and Publication Types

Index Terms

Clinical assessment tools (can be exploded)
Comparative studies
Diagnosis (can be exploded)
Diagnosis, cardiovascular (can be exploded)

Diagnosis, computer assisted (can be exploded)
Diagnosis, delayed
Diagnosis, developmental (can be exploded)
Diagnosis, differential
Diagnosis, digestive system (can be exploded)
Diagnosis, dual (psychiatry)
Diagnosis, endocrine (can be exploded)
Diagnosis, eye (can be exploded)
Diagnosis, laboratory (can be exploded)
Diagnosis, musculoskeletal (can be exploded)
Diagnosis, neurologic (can be exploded)
Diagnosis, ob-gyn (can be exploded)
Diagnosis, oral (can be exploded)
Diagnosis, otorhinolaryngologic (can be exploded)
Diagnosis, psychosocial (can be exploded)
Diagnosis, radioisotope (can be exploded)
Diagnosis, respiratory system (can be exploded)
Diagnosis, surgical (can be exploded)
Diagnosis, urologic (can be exploded)
Diagnostic errors (can be exploded)
Diagnostic imaging (can be exploded)
Diagnostic reasoning
Diagnostic tests, routine
False negative results
False positive results
Genetic screening
Health screening (can be exploded)
Mandatory testing
Maximum likelihood
Measurement issues and assessments (can be exploded)
Nursing assessment
Nursing diagnosis
Observer bias (can be exploded)
Odds ratio
Precision
Predictive value of tests
Probability
Reproducibility of results
Sensitivity and specificity
Substance abuse detection (can be exploded)
Validity (can be exploded)
Vision screening

Subheadings

Diagnosis
Radiography
Ultrasonography
Diagnostic use
Nursing
Symptoms

Publication Types

Diagnostic images

EMBASE

Index Terms, Subheadings, and Publication Types

Index Terms

Accuracy
Area under the curve
Bayes theorem
Classification (can be exploded)
Coding and classification (can be exploded)
Computer assisted diagnosis (can be exploded)
Diagnosis (can be exploded)
Diagnostic accuracy
Diagnostic error
Diagnostic procedure (can be exploded)
Diagnostic test (can be exploded)
Diagnostic value
Differential diagnosis
Discriminant analysis
Disease classification (can be exploded)
Genetic screening
Laboratory diagnosis (can be exploded)
Mass screening (can be exploded)
Maximum likelihood method
Newborn screening
Nomogram
Observer variation
Pharmacokinetics (can be exploded)
Probability
Psychiatric diagnosis (can be exploded)

Receiver operating characteristic
Screening test
Sensitivity and specificity
Screening (can be exploded)
Substance abuse
Thorax radiography
Vision test (can be exploded)
Visual system examination (can be exploded)

Subheadings

Diagnosis
Diagnostic use

Publication Types

None

PsycINFO

Index Terms, Subheadings, and Publication Types

Index Terms

Computer Assisted Diagnosis (can be exploded)
Criterion referenced test
Diagnosis (can be exploded)
Differential diagnosis
Dual diagnosis
Health screening (can be exploded)
Medical diagnosis (can be exploded)
Misdiagnosis
Neuropsychological assessment (can be exploded)
Prenatal diagnosis
Probability (can be exploded)
Psychodiagnosis (can be exploded)
Psychodiagnostic interview (can be exploded)
Psychodiagnostic typologies (can be exploded)
Psychological screening inventory
Screening tests (can be exploded)
Screening (can be exploded)
Statistical probability (can be exploded)
Symptom checklists
Taxonomies

Subheadings

None

Publication Types

None

EXAMPLES OF TEXTWORDS AND INDEXING USING OUR CLINICAL EXAMPLE

Citation for Our Clinical Example

Duer A, Østergaard M, Hørslev-Petersen K, Vallø J. Magnetic resonance imaging and bone scintigraphy in the differential diagnosis of unclassified arthritis. Ann Rheum Dis. 2008;67:48–51.

Textwords and Index Terms Used in Our Clinical Example

Textwords (in the Title and Abstract of the Article)

Diagnos:
Differential diagnosis
Specificit:

MEDLINE INDEXING

Diagnosis (subheading)
Diagnosis, differential
Diagnostic use (subheading)
Sensitivity and specificity

EMBASE INDEXING

Diagnosis (subheading)
Differential diagnosis
Disease classification

LINKS TO OTHER RESOURCES

Link to how to use an article about differential diagnosis: http://www.cche.net/usersguides/probability.asp

Link to how to use an article about disease manifestation:http://www.cche.net/usersguides/manifestations.asp

EXERCISES

Note that the search possibilities (answers) are detailed in the Appendix.

1. What is the differential diagnosis for unexplained drop attacks in older persons?
2. What is the clinical manifestation of Lyme disease in children?

REFERENCES

1. Burbige EJ, Huang SH, Bayless TM. Clinical manifestations of Crohn's disease in children and adolescents. *Pediatrics.* 1975;55:866–71.
2. Duer A, Østergaard M, Hørslev-Petersen K, Vallø J. Magnetic resonance imaging and bone scintigraphy in the differential diagnosis of unclassified arthritis. *Ann Rheum Dis.* 2008;67:48–51.
3. Guyatt G, Rennie D, Meade MO, Cook DJ. *Users' Guide to the Medical Literature. A Manual for Evidence-Based Clinical Practice.* 2 ed. New York, NY: McGraw-Hill Companies Inc, 2002; 399–417.
4. Richardson WS, Glasziou P, Polashenski WA, Wilson MC. A new arrival: evidence about differential diagnosis. *ACP J Club. 2000;133:A11–12.*

9

Qualitative Studies

Susan Marks and Nancy Wilczynski

INTRODUCTION

Up to this point, the study designs that we have described (e.g., randomized controlled trial, cohort study, case-control study) have been what are called **quantitative** studies. Quantitative study designs are most appropriate when answering questions of "how many" or "how much." For example, if you want to find out whether guided imagery could reduce pain in children with leukemia, you should look for a randomized controlled trial in which children are randomly allocated to participate in interactive guided imagery sessions (experimental group) or to an equal amount of time simply visiting with a volunteer (control group). After each visit, the 2 groups are compared to see how many children in each group report reductions in pain. Some types of research or clinical questions, however, are best answered using another type of study design called **qualitative**. When you want to know about how people *feel* or *experience* certain situations, a qualitative study is usually a better choice. If you wanted to understand, for example, how the families of children diagnosed with cancer learned to cope with the diagnosis and the changes it brought to their lives, a qualitative study would be more likely to provide meaningful information. In such a study, a researcher might hold in-depth interviews with parents of children with cancer, beginning with a general statement, such as, "Tell me what it was like to find out that your child had cancer." The researcher would then systematically analyze verbatim transcripts of the interviews, looking for common themes and connections among them to describe the experience of parents coping with a child's diagnosis of cancer.

To better understand what qualitative research is all about, it may be helpful to see how it differs from quantitative research. The purpose of this comparison is not to determine which method is "better." Quantitative study designs have a long history in the health care literature, whereas qualitative studies are relatively new. Proponents of both quantitative and qualitative research have debated the relative merits and weaknesses of each, but we feel that both methods have a place in health care research. The most important thing is to look for the type of study design that can provide the best answers to your questions—and how we define "best" can also vary, according to the question asked. Qualitative studies usually differ from quantitative studies in terms of the type of questions they address, how samples are chosen, methods of data collection and analysis, and how results are presented. As well, the terminology used in reports of qualitative studies sometimes differs. For example, those who are studied are often called participants rather than patients or subjects, and the study results are referred to as findings. The general differences are summarized in Table 9–1, and some of the key points will be illustrated in the clinical example given in the next section.

CLINICAL EXAMPLE

Jones and colleagues conducted a study to better understand the reasons for nonadherence to cardiac rehabilitation programs.[1] This qualitative study included 49 patients participating in the Birmingham Rehabilitation Uptake Maximisation (BRUM) study, a randomized controlled trial that compared home-based and hospital-based cardiac rehabilitation after myocardial infarction or revascularization. Trial nurses provided the names of patients who had not adhered to their rehabilitation program. These patients were contacted and asked if they were willing to be interviewed about the cardiac rehabilitation program. Forty-nine patients participated in individual, recorded, semi-structured interviews that addressed topics related to the patients' cardiac events, including their expectations and experiences of their rehabilitation programs and lifestyle changes. The content of later interviews was revised to address issues emerging from earlier interviews. Transcripts were read independently by 3 investigators, and the main themes and subthemes were identified and agreed on.

The reasons for nonadherence were grouped into categories, and repeated readings of the transcripts and field notes also enabled identification of a crucial or critical reason among those patients who had given more than 1 reason for nonadherence. Four categories of nonadherence were identified.

1. *Alternative exercise and activities.* Although participants did not adhere to their cardiac rehabilitation program, they exercised in other ways that better fit with their lifestyles.
2. *Other health problems.* Many participants had other health problems that affected their ability to participate in their cardiac rehabilitation program. They perceived these health problems as bigger barriers to exercising than their heart condition.

Table 9–1

Common Features of Qualitative and Quantitative Studies

Features	Qualitative Studies	Quantitative Studies
Type of question	Most appropriate for questions about meaning and how people feel and experience situations.	Most appropriate for questions of "how many" (patients get better) or "how much" (do they get better).
Sampling	Theoretical or purposeful sampling of a relatively small number of people who have in-depth knowledge or experience of the topic of interest. The goal is to learn about people in a specific context and not to generate findings that will be applicable to a wide variety of people. Although there may be few participants, there are many "sampling units" of textual data generated from each participant.	Probability sampling to ensure that the sample is representative of a more general population and to minimize bias. The goal is to ensure that the findings will be generalizable to general populations of people. Large sample sizes are often needed.
Data collection	Data collection often involves unstructured interviews although other methods are also used (e.g., observation of people in natural settings and focus groups). Responses given in interviews with the first few participants may lead to modifications in how later interviews are conducted (iterative approach).	Systematic data collection using structured formats. Blinding of data collectors or participants is sometimes necessary to avoid biasing results.
Analysis	Data analysis takes place concurrent with the data collection process, and is ongoing. Units of analysis are thoughts or concepts, which are classified into categories or themes.	Units of analysis are people (e.g., number of elderly people who have fallen), events (e.g., number of falls), or test scores, etc., which are counted or measured in some way. The numbers are combined and manipulated using statistical tests.
Presentation of findings	Rich, detailed findings are presented in narrative format, sometimes accompanied by diagrams of theoretical models. Many direct quotations are included.	Findings pertaining to the sample or specific sub-samples are summarized in terms of numerical relations or statistics.

3. *Personal reasons.* Some people could not attend hospital-based cardiac rehabilitation programs because they had to care for others who could not be left alone for long periods.

4. *Program-related changes.* Many participants in the home-based cardiac rehabilitation program felt that lack of motivation was the main reason for non-adherence.

METHODOLOGICAL ISSUES

This example illustrates several features common to many qualitative studies:

- The **research question** focused on the experiences of a particular group of people in a particular context (i.e., the experiences of patients who participated in, but did not adhere to, 1 of 2 cardiac rehabilitation programs after myocardial infarction or revascularization).

- Selection of the **study sample** was *purposeful.* The intent was to select the participants best able to meet the informational needs of the study.[2] Therefore, it was important to select participants who had not adhered to the program. A sample size was not identified ahead of time. The study investigator included all patients who consented to participate.

- **Data collection and analysis** occurred concurrently and influenced the next step of the research process. For example, immediately after the interview with the first participant, the researcher will analyze the data, beginning with the identification and classification of words and thoughts into common themes and categories. This analysis may lead the researcher to slightly modify the questions that will be posed to the second participant. Similarly, after the second interview, the researcher will examine the data to see what does and does not fit into themes or categories identified from the first interview, and whether additional refinements or categories are warranted. This process continues until data saturation occurs (i.e., until the researcher is no longer hearing or seeing new information). In the example, interviews were scheduled to include issues emerging from previous interviews. Data were also collected using different methods. Interview transcripts were the primary data source, but field notes made by the researcher provided additional, complementary data on participants' nonverbal behaviors and activity levels.

- The **unit of analysis** was words or concepts, rather than people or events as in quantitative studies. In the example, transcripts were read independently by 3 investigators, and the main themes and subthemes were identified and agreed upon. The reasons for nonadherence were grouped into categories, and repeated readings of the transcripts and field notes also enabled identification of a single crucial or critical reason among patients who had given more than 1 reason for nonadherence.

- The **study findings** were presented in a narrative format, with numerous examples of *verbatim statements* made by participants. For example, to illustrate some of the reasons for nonadherence, the following quotations were presented: "…we've been too busy doing the decorating and the garden. I haven't had the chance to go out walking. But as I say I'm not still…"; "…they wanted me to go up to the hospital at nighttime. I said, I'm sorry, I'm not being awkward, but I don't go out at nighttime." These examples help the reader to see how the researcher arrived at certain themes. In some cases, the researcher may develop a model or theory that attempts to explain processes or how different themes are interrelated. Reports of qualitative studies can be quite lengthy, restricted only by the word limits of the publishing journal. Indeed, many authors of qualitative reports find it difficult to convey the depth and richness of the data they have collected in the limited space available in most journals. Similarly, the above summary is only a superficial description of the findings of Jones and colleagues to give readers a flavor of qualitative research.

Methodological Approaches

Both qualitative researchers and readers of qualitative studies alike may encounter difficulties when trying to categorize or assess such research by "type." The specific interests and intentions of the originators of qualitative methodological traditions, such as phenomenology or grounded theory, are often quite different from those of qualitative researchers working in applied health fields.[3] Researchers often "violate" these methodological traditions by applying only selected aspects of the methods that are relevant to their own interests.[3] For example, researchers may label their study design as "phenomenology," but, in practice, they "violate" the tradition by going beyond the intent of phenomenology (which is to simply present what people experience or feel at the deepest levels) and develop explanatory or interpretive models of the findings.[3] In fact, some nursing researchers have proposed terms such as "interpretive description"[3] and "qualitative description"[4] to reflect the important type of qualitative research that nurses actually do. Sandelowski[4] refers to "qualitative descriptive studies," which aim to provide "a comprehensive summary of an event in the everyday terms of those events" (p 336). The designs of such studies are an eclectic, but considered, combination of sampling, data collection, analysis, and presentation techniques.

Rather than provide a comprehensive typology of qualitative studies, we will instead describe 3 of the more common methodological approaches that inform qualitative studies: phenomenology, grounded theory, and ethnography. These 3 qualitative methods aim to describe the complexity of human experiences in context.[5]

Phenomenology is concerned with describing the human or "lived" experience using the subjective or first-person experience as a source of knowledge. It is often used when little is known about a topic.[6] Palese and colleagues[7] did a phenomenology study to describe the experiences of 21 patients with brain tumors before, during, and after awake craniotomy, a surgical procedure done under local anesthesia—that is, patients are awake during the procedure. They interact with the neurosurgeon during the procedure as different parts of the brain are stimulated. Patients participated in individual interviews the day before surgery and the day after surgery. Each interview lasted 30 to 60 minutes and was guided by open-ended questions such as "Please tell me how you feel now, waiting for this operation ..." and "What do you remember about your intraoperative experience?" Patients' concerns before, during, and after the surgery were described. Before surgery, patients were focused on self-preservation; they felt that having the surgery under local anesthesia was not negotiable because it was a way to prevent disabilities during tumor removal. They also focused on working out their role during surgery and preparing to do what the neurosurgeon asked them to do. They feared being unable to control their actions during surgery. During surgery, patients were concerned with keeping the situation under control. They concentrated on what others were doing in the operating room, anxiously awaiting to be asked to perform their first task. Patients tried to imagine what was happening during each stage of the surgery so that they could remain in control of the situation. Speaking to the neurosurgeon and receiving feedback and listening to staff talk to each other were reassuring to patients. After surgery, patients were intent on reassuring themselves and others, taking stock of any language and motor disabilities. The overall experience of awake craniotomy was described by patients using metaphors, such as "an out of this world experience" and "touching the sun with my hands."

Grounded theory studies are designed, as the name suggests, to develop theory grounded in the real world of the participants. Thus, in addition to describing phenomena, grounded theory studies attempt to explain them.[8] A good example of grounded theory is a study by Schreiber[9] on the process of women's recovery from depression. Twenty women who had recovered from depression participated in interviews lasting about 90 minutes. Interview transcripts were analyzed using constant comparative analysis. A theory emerged that explained the 6-stage process of "(re)defining my self" that the women went through as they recovered from depression:(1) "My self before" referred to a time before depression, (2) seeing the abyss, (3) telling my story, (4) seeking understanding, (5) cluing in, and (6) seeing with clarity

Ethnographic studies seek to learn about how people interpret their experience and adapt their behavior within the context of their own culturally defined environment.[10] A good example is a study done by

Tourigny[11] involving 6 African American youths who had deliberately exposed themselves to HIV. All of the participants were HIV positive, and had at least 1 family member with HIV infection or AIDS. Tourigny met with these youths over time, with meetings often taking place in the respondents' homes while they carried on with activities such as washing dishes, caring for family members, or keeping watch over gang-related traffic in their neighborhoods. The stories of each of the youths and why they deliberately sought exposure to HIV were presented in a narrative format, with many direct quotes. For example, Brendon's story began as follows:

> Brendon was 22 when we met. A man of courtly manners and a gentle presence, he would cry at any mention of his 40-year-old sister, Debra—her illness, her sex work, her drug habit, and, particularly her children: his niece, a healthy 8-year-old, and his 5-year-old AIDS-afflicted nephew. {....} After more than 3 years of unemployment, friendships with people who are still working gradually offered little but embarrassment. His own despair eroded his emotional resilience; his easy smile became frozen, and he started talking about wanting to die. One hot afternoon, Brendon looked over my shoulder as he said, "Yo...doc, I got it too. Everybody was raggin' me about not getting nowhere, not getting no job, not doing nothing. Well there ain't nothing to do here. I looked at my sister, and she got everybody seeing to her hand and foot and she ain't even sick. This AIDS things don't need make you sick at all, but people sure listen up when you talk. She's getting good money from the feds...." (p 155)

Tournigy interpreted these stories in the context of the social inequalities of inner city life. She found that the youths were overwhelmed by worry, depression, caregiving, and hopelessness, and robbed of their childhood by poverty. They were deeply involved with their loved ones, and therefore leaving was not an alternative. With no other obvious recourse, AIDS offered a way to access care and resources.

Synthesis of Qualitative Studies

The findings of multiple qualitative studies on a specific topic are sometimes combined and analyzed. Such syntheses differ from typical quantitative systematic reviews in their intent to integrate, rather than simply aggregate, the findings of individual studies.[12] Some of the terms commonly used to describe methods of aggregating qualitative research include **qualitative meta-analysis, meta-summary, meta-synthesis**, and **meta-ethnography.**[12-15]

SUMMARY

Qualitative studies generally differ from quantitative studies, such as randomized controlled trials or cohort studies, in terms of the type of question asked, sample selection, data collection and analysis, and reporting of results. Qualitative studies provide the most relevant information when the goal is to know how people feel or experience certain situations. The number of people sampled is usually much smaller than for quantitative studies, and participants are often selected on the basis of their knowledge or experience of the content area. Common methods of data collection include in-depth unstructured interviews, focus groups, observation, and use of print records, such as diaries or historical accounts. Whereas the unit of analysis in quantitative studies is primarily people or events, the unit of analysis in qualitative studies is a thought or a concept. Study findings are presented in the form of rich, detailed narratives that describe common themes and understandings, or sometimes as diagrams that depict how different themes are interrelated.

SEARCHING METHODOLOGY

Now that we have summarized the components of qualitative studies, we move onto searching for qualitative studies in the large electronic databases such as MEDLINE. This task can be challenging, but using search terms that target the methodology specific to qualitative studies in addition to your content terms (e.g., depression) can aid in retrieval effectiveness. The search terms available for use in 4 large electronic databases are listed below. The terms were compiled during the Clinical Hedges Study[16] based on input from clinicians and librarians in the United States and Canada. Index terms, subheadings, and publication types are assigned to each article in the database by staff working for the electronic database (e.g., MEDLINE). Textwords are used to search for articles using the article title and the article abstract. The Clinical Hedges Study developed search strategies for detecting qualitative studies in MEDLINE, CINAHL, EMBASE, and PsycINFO; preferred search terms for these 4 databases are summarized below.

MEDLINE

MeSH, Subheadings, Publication Types, and Textwords

MeSH (Medical Subject Headings — Index Terms)

Interviews as topic* (can be exploded)
Health services administration (can be exploded)*

Anecdotes

---

*Indicates a preferred term as determined in the Clinical Hedges Study.[17]

Attitude to health (can be exploded)
Clinical nursing research
Evaluation studies
Focus groups
Knowledge, attitudes, practice
Observation
Nursing administration research
Nursing education research
Nursing evaluation research
Nursing methodology research
Nursing research (can be exploded)
Nursing theory
Tape recording (can be exploded)
Videotape recording

Subheadings

Psychology*

Publication Types

Interview

Textwords (Same List Is Used for All 4 Databases)

Experience*
Interview:*
Qualitative*
Qualitative study*
Themes*

Analytic memo:
Anecdote:
Audiotape:
Audiotape: interview:
Axial coding
Central themes
Colaizzi
Conceptual categories
Conceptual framework
Concurrent analys:
Concurrent data analys:
Concurrent data collection:

*Indicates a preferred term as determined in the Clinical Hedges Study.[17-20]

Confirmability
Content analys:
Constant comparative analys:
Constant comparative method
Convenience sampl:
Data saturation
Dependability
Descriptive analys:
Document analys:
Emergent theor:
Emic
Ethnographic method:
Ethnographic research
Ethnographic stud:
Ethnographic theme:
Ethnography
Ethnological research
Ethnomethodology
Ethnonursing research
Etic
Exploratory interview:
Exploratory design
Face to face interview:
Field notes
Field observation:
Focus group:
Focused interview:
Giorgi
Glaser and Strauss
Grounded theory
Heidegger
Hermeneutic
Husserl
In-depth interview:
Indepth interview:
In-depth observation:
Indepth observation:
Inductive:
Inductive analys:
Inductive grounded approach
Inductive reasoning
Informational redundancy
Iterative approach
Interpretive:

Interpretive analys:
Interpretive anthropology
Interpretive method
Interview guide:
Life experience:
Life histor:
Lived experience:
Maximum variation sampling
Merleau
Merleau-Ponty
Meta-ethnography
Metaethnography
Meta-narratives
Metanarratives
Narrative:
Narrative analys:
Narrative format:
Naturalistic:
Naturalistic inquiry
Naturalistic stud:
Nonparticipant observation:
Observation:
Observational method:
Open-ended
Open coding
Participant observation:
Phenomen:
Phenomenological:
Phenomenological research
Phenomenology
Probability sampling
Purposeful sampling
Purposive sample
Purposive sampling
Qualitative stud:
Qualitative analys:
Qualitative validity
Record: observation:
Ricoeur
Saturation
Selective coding
Semistructured
Semi-structured
Semistructured interview:

Semi-structured interview:
Snowball sampling
Spiegelberg
Stratified purposeful sampling
Symbolic interactionism
Tape record:
Ttaped discussion:
Telephone interview:
Thematic analys:
Thematic content analys:
Thematic content
Theoretical:
Theoretical grounding
Theoretical sample:
Theoretical sample model:
Theoretical sampling
Theoretical saturation
Transcendental phenomenology
Transcrib:
Transcrib: verbatim
Transcript:
Transcription
Triangulation
Unstructured interview:
Van Kaam
Van Manen
Verbatim
Verbatim statement:
Videotap:
Videotape: recording:

CINAHL (CUMULATIVE INDEX TO NURSING AND ALLIED HEALTH LITERATURE)

Index Terms, Subheadings, and Publication Types

Index Terms

Attitude (can be exploded)*
Audiorecording*
Interviews (can be exploded)*
Grounded theory*

---

*Indicates a preferred term as determined in the Clinical Hedges Study.[18]

Qualitative studies*
Study design (can be exploded)*
Thematic analysis*

Attitude to abortion
Attitude to aging
Attitude to AIDS
Attitude to breast feeding
Attitude to change
Attitude to death (can be exploded)
Attitude to health (can be exploded)
Attitude of health personnel (can be exploded)
Attitude to illness (can be exploded)
Attitude to life
Attitude to mental illness
Attitude to pregnancy
Attitude to sexuality (can be exploded)
Clinical nursing research
Clinical research (can be exploded)
Cluster sample
Conceptual framework
"Confirmability (research)"
Constant comparative method
Content analysis
Convenience sample
Conversation
"Credibility (research)"
Critical theory
"Dependability (research)"
Descriptive research
Descriptive statistics
Discourse analysis
"Education, nursing, research based"
Ethnographic research
Ethnography
Ethnological research
Ethnonursing research
Evaluation research (can be exploded)
Exploratory research
Family attitudes (can be exploded)
Field studies
Focus groups

*Indicates a preferred term as determined in the Clinical Hedges Study.[18]

Formative evaluation research
Life experiences (can be exploded)
Life histories
Narratives
Naturalistic inquiry
Nonparticipant observation
Nonprobability sample (can be exploded)
Nursing administration research
Nursing knowledge
"Nursing models, theoretical"
Nursing theory (can be exploded)
Observation (can be exploded)
Observational methods (can be exploded)
Parental attitudes
Participant observation
Patient attitudes
Patient satisfaction
Personal satisfaction (can be exploded)
Phenomenological research
Phenomenology
Probability sample
Purposive sample
Qualitative validity (can be exploded)
Quota sample
Research nursing
Semi-structured interview
Snowball sample
Social attitudes
Sociological theory (can be exploded)
Structured categories
Structured interview
Suicide ideation
Summative evaluation research
Theoretical sample
Transferability
Triangulation
Unstructured categories
Unstructured interview
Videorecording

Subheadings

None

Publication Types

None

EMBASE

Index Terms, Subheadings, and Publication Types

Index Terms

Health care facilities and services (can be exploded)*
Health care organization (can be exploded)*
Interview*

Analytic method
Attitude
Clinical observation
Concept formation
Experience
Information processing (can be exploded)
Life event
Literature
Nursing education
Nursing (can be exploded)
Observation
Patient attitude
Qualitative analysis
Symbolism
Tape recorder
Theoretical study
Videorecording
Videotape

Subheadings

None

Publication Types

None

*Indicates a preferred term as determined in the Clinical Hedges Study.[19]

PsycINFO

Index Terms, Subheadings, and Publication Types

Index Terms

Content analysis (can be exploded)
Credibility
Discourse analysis
Ethnography
Grounded Theory (added in 2003)
Health attitudes
Hermeneutics
Interviews (can be exploded)
Life experiences
Narratives
Observation methods
Phenomenology
Qualitative research (added in 2003)
Symbolic interactionism
Tape recorders (can be exploded)
Theoretical interpretations
Videotape recorders

Subheadings

None

Publication Types

None

EXAMPLES OF TEXTWORDS AND INDEXING USING OUR CLINICAL EXAMPLE

Citation for Our Clinical Example

Jones M, Jolly K, Raftery J, et al. "DNA" may not mean "did not participate": a qualitative study of reasons for non-adherence at home- and centre-based cardiac rehabilitation. *Fam Pract*. 2007;24:343–357.

Textwords and Index Terms Used in Our Clinical Example

Textwords (in the Title and Abstract of the Article)

Interview:*
Qualitative*
Qualitative study*

MEDLINE INDEXING

Interview as topic*

Attitude to health

CINAHL INDEXING

Journal not indexed in CINAHL

EMBASE INDEXING

Patient attitude
Qualitative analysis

PsycINFO INDEXING

None of the identified terms

PROVEN STRATEGIES

Search Strategies (Filters) Derived during the Clinical Hedges Study[17-20]

Filter*	Medline (Ovid syntax)	CINAHL† (Ovid syntax)	EMBASE (Ovid syntax)	PsycINFO (Ovid syntax)
Sensitive	interview:.tw. OR px.fs. OR exp health services administration	exp study design OR exp attitude OR exp interviews	interview:.tw. OR qualitative. tw. OR health care organization	experience:.mp. OR interview:. tw. OR qualitative:. tw.

Continued

*Indicates a preferred term as determined in the Clinical Hedges Study.[17-20]

Filter*	Medline (Ovid syntax)	CINAHL† (Ovid syntax)	EMBASE (Ovid syntax)	PsycINFO (Ovid syntax)
Specific	qualitative.tw. OR themes.tw.	grounded theory.sh. OR thematic analysis.mp.	qualitative.tw. OR qualitative study.tw.	qualitative:.tw. OR themes.tw.
Minimize difference between Sensitivity and Specificity	interview:.mp. OR experience:.mp. OR qualitative.tw.	interview.tw. OR audiorecord-ing.sh. OR qualitative stud:.mp.	interview:.tw. OR exp health care organization OR experiences.tw.	experiences.tw. OR interview:.tw. OR qualitative.tw.

*See the Introduction for a description of how to use these filters and where to find them in Ovid and PubMed.

†In 2009 CINAHL will only be offered through EBSCO. The CINAHL search strategies have been translated and are available for use in EBSCO.

LINKS TO OTHER RESOURCES

Link to information regarding the Clinical Hedges Study: http://hiru.mc-master.ca/hiru/HIRU_Hedges_home.aspx

Link to How to use an article of a qualitative nature: http://www.cche.net/usersguides/qualitative.asp

EXERCISES

Note that the search possibilities (answers) are detailed in the Appendix.

1. What are the experiences of inpatients who have pressure ulcers?
2. What are the perceptions of patients and health care providers regarding communicating about sexuality and intimacy after a cancer diagnosis?

REFERENCES

1. Jones M, Jolly K, Raftery J, et al. 'DNA' may not mean 'did not participate': a qualitative study of reasons for non-adherence at home- and centre-based cardiac rehabilitation. *Fam Pract.* 2007;24:343-357.
2. Thompson C. If you could just provide me with a sample: examining sampling in qualitative and quantitative research papers. *Evidence-Based Nursing.* 1999;2:68-70.

3. Thorne S, Kirkham SR, MacDonald-Emes J. Interpretive description: a non-categorical qualitative alternative for developing nursing knowledge. *Res Nurs Health.* 1997;20:169-177.

4. Sandelowski M. Whatever happened to qualitative description? *Res Nurs Health.* 2000;23:334-340.

5. Ploeg J. Identifying the best research design to fit the question. Part 2: qualitative designs. *Evidence-Based Nursing.* 1999;2:36-37.

6. Smith BA. The problem drinker's lived experience of suffering: an exploration using hermeneutic phenomenology. *J Adv Nurs.* 1998;27:213–222.

7. Palese A, Skrap M, Fachin M, et al. The experience of patients undergoing awake craniotomy: in the patients' own words. A qualitative study. *Cancer Nurs.* 2008;31:166-172.

8. Corbin J, Strauss A. Grounded theory research: procedures, canons, and evaluative criteria. *Qual Sociol.* 1990;13:3-21.

9. Schreiber R. (Re)defining my self: women's process of recovery from depression. *Qual Health Res.* 1996;6:469-491.

10. Aamodt AM. Ethnography and epistemology: generating nursing knowledge In: Morse JM, ed. *Qualitative Nursing Research: A Contemporary Dialogue.* Newbury Park, CA: Sage Publications, 1991; 40-53.

11. Tourigny SC. Some new dying trick: African-American youths "choosing" HIV/AIDS. *Qual Health Res.* 1998;8:149-167.

12. Walsh D, Downe S. Meta-synthesis method for qualitative research: a literature review. *J Adv Nurs.* 2005;50:204-211.

13. Patterson BL, Thorne SE, Canam C, et al. *Meta-Study of Qualitative Research. A Practical Guide to Meta-Analysis and Metasynthesis.* Thousand Oaks, CA: Sage; 2001.

14. Bondas T, Hall EO. Challenges in approaching metasynthesis research. *Qual Health Res.* 2007;17:113-121.

15. Atkins S, Lewin S, Smith H. Conducting a meta-ethnography of qualitative literature: lessons learnt. *BMC Med Res Methodol.* 2008;8:21

16. Wilczynski NL, Morgan D, Haynes RB; Hedges Team. An overview of the design and methods for retrieving high-quality studies for clinical care. *BMC Med Inform Decis Mak.* 2005;5:20.

17. Wong SS, Wilczynski NL, Haynes RB; Hedges Team. Developing optimal search strategies for detecting clinically relevant qualitative studies in MEDLINE. *Medinfo.* 2004;11(Pt 1):311-316.

18. Wilczynski NL, Marks S, Haynes RB. Search strategies for identifying qualitative studies in CINAHL. *Qual Health Res.* 2007;17:705-710.

19. Walters LA, Wilczynski NL, Haynes RB; Hedges Team. Developing optimal search strategies for retrieving clinically relevant qualitative studies in EMBASE. *Qual Health Res.* 2006;16:162-168.

20. McKibbon KA, Wilczynski NL, Haynes RB. Developing optimal search strategies for retrieving qualitative studies in PsycINFO. *Eval Health Prof.* 2006;29:440-454.

ASSESSING THE QUALITY OF QUALITATIVE STUDIES

Various authors have proposed criteria to assess the quality of qualitative research; others have argued against the use of such criteria. Selected citations are provided below as examples.

- Campbell R, Pound P, Pope C, et al. Evaluating meta-ethnography: a synthesis of qualitative research on lay experiences of diabetes and diabetes care. *Soc Sci Med.* 2003;56:671-684.
- Daly J, Willis K, Small R, Green J, et al. A hierarchy of evidence for assessing qualitative health research. *J Clin Epidemiol.* 2007;60:43-49.
- Giacomini MK, Cook DJ, for the Evidence-Based Medicine Working Group. Users' guides to the medical literature XXIII. Qualitative research in health care. A. Are the results of the study valid? *JAMA.* 2000;284:357-362.
- Giacomini MK, Cook DJ, for the Evidence-Based Medicine Working Group. Users' guides to the medical literature XXIII. Qualitative research in health care. B. What are the results and how do they help me care for my patients? *JAMA.* 2000;284:478-482.
- Rolfe G. Validity, trustworthiness and rigour: quality and the idea of qualitative research. *J Adv Nurs.* 2006;53:304-310.

Secondary Publications: Systematic Review Articles

Ann McKibbon

We have completed our summary of the primary EBHC studies of therapy, diagnosis, etiology and causation, natural history and prognosis, clinical prediction guides, decision analyses, differential diagnosis and disease manifestation, and qualitative studies. The order in which we considered these 8 categories reflects their respective prevalence in the health care literature. Qualitative studies, like quantitative methods, have many different tools and techniques that can be used to answer important questions. Qualitative studies answer the "how" and "why" questions while the quantitative studies answer "what," "when," "where," "how many," and "how much" questions.

To complete our understanding of the types of evidence most useful to EBHC practitioners, we turn to **secondary publications**. They are called "secondary" because researchers take data from previously published or unpublished studies, summarize and analyze the combined results, draw conclusions, and publish their resulting new knowledge in these publications. The secondary publications are systematic reviews that include meta-analyses, clinical practice guidelines, economic analyses, and health technology assessment reports.

Secondary publications can synthesize qualitative and quantitative data. More quantitative than qualitative secondary analyses studies exist reflecting the relative numbers of primary publications of qualitative and quantitative studies. Many clinicians and researchers believe that a synthesis of several original studies provides better, more powerful evidence with greater potential influence on clinical decisions than a single study. Many people start their searches for evidence to support their EBHC quests with a strategy to retrieve a systematic review or another secondary publication. This chapter will concentrate on systematic reviews and meta-analyses. Subsequent chapters will address the other 3 secondary publications:

clinical practice guidelines, economics studies, and health technology assessment reports.

SYSTEMATIC REVIEW ARTICLES AND META-ANALYSES

Evidence-based health care has embraced and further developed a new type of review article, called a **systematic review article.** Conventional review articles are often designated as **narrative reviews** to differentiate them from systematic review articles. Systematic reviews differ from narrative reviews on at least 2 major points. A systematic review article is based explicitly on a careful collection, review, and evaluation of the evidence on a topic, rather than being just a summary of knowledge by an individual who has some background in the area. These experts may include strong evidence in their narrative reviews but this evidence is often mixed inextricably with opinion.

Narrative review articles have been equated with textbook chapters that broadly summarize a topic and present it in a narrative format. These reviews can, but often do not, include numerical, statistical, or other cross-study analyses that synthesize the findings of original studies and come to an evidence-based "bottom line" or conclusion. Because of their textbook chapter-like format and content, traditional review articles are often more useful for understanding a new or complex topic. Students appreciate traditional or narrative review articles because they are vehicles that summarize broad topic areas. The *New England Journal of Medicine* publishes many narrative reviews. Reviews in 3 consecutive issues in July 2008 covered topics of initial management of epilepsy,[1] acetylcysteine for acetaminophen poisoning,[2] and hypoparathroidism.[3] All 3 topics are broad.

Systematic reviews are often more clinically based, with the purpose of answering a narrower and more focused clinical topic, such as: What is the effectiveness (i.e., do they work in the "real" world) and safety shown across randomized controlled trials of beta-interferon to prevent relapses in multiple sclerosis?

To be considered a systematic review article, it must first clearly state why the review is being done: the purpose. For example, Jepson and Craig[4] completed a systematic review with the explicit purpose of evaluating whether cranberry juice or concentrate in tablet form reduced the number of urinary tract infections in middle-aged women. This requirement of having an explicit statement of purpose is similar to primary studies, in that any study must define and establish the research question before the research starts. Jepson and Craig combined data from 10 studies (1049 women) and found that cranberries reduced the number of urinary tract infections by approximately 40% (RR 0.61, 95% CI 0.40 to 0.91).

Moreover, the methods used to find the primary studies to be included (e.g., search strategies, review of bibliographies of other review articles, or contact with the authors of important, relevant studies) must be described. To illustrate this, the following description of the retrieval process was included by van Sleuwen and colleagues [5] in their systematic review article on the effectiveness of swaddling babies:

> **Electronic searches were conducted in PubMed (1966 to February 2007), PsycINFO (1887 to February 2007), EMBASE (1974 to February 2007), the Cochrane library (2007, Issue 1), and Blackwell Synergy (1990 to February 2007). We used the Medical Subject Headings (MeSH) heading swaddling. Manually searched reference lists were used also.**

In addition to stating searching methods, the authors of systematic reviews should also state the inclusion and exclusion criteria used to select articles for inclusion in their review. These criteria should be detailed enough so that anyone could replicate them. van Sleuwen et al [5] stated:

> **All published randomized, controlled trials (RCTs) that evaluated the intervention of swaddling were included, as were all other studies on swaddling in relation to sleep state and arousal, temperature control, motor development, SIDS, (acute) respiratory infections, bone development, DDH [developmental dysplasia of the hip], pain control, the effect on crying behavior, and breastfeeding and neonatal weight loss.**

Although some librarians may question the use of "MeSH headings" for EMBASE searches and the use of only 1 term in the strategy, at least the search could be easily replicated. With provision of the search strategy information and the inclusion and exclusion criteria we can, if we choose, replicate the search process and examine the evidence (original studies) that the authors used to analyze, draw their conclusions, and make recommendations. The searching information can also be used to update the data and findings in the article and provide templates for other searchers interested in the same or a similar topic. Without the search strategy and inclusion/exclusion information, we cannot distinguish if the authors are providing hard evidence or speculation and opinion.

The authors concluded that swaddling has both benefits and some problems after their review of data from 9 randomized controlled trials. Infants who are swaddled sleep longer and are less prone to being aroused from sleep—news that most new mothers might appreciate.

HISTORY OF SYSTEMATIC REVIEW ARTICLES

The systematic review methodology was developed and refined in the disciplines of education and psychology in the late 1960s and early 1970s, although some early examples exist in the health care literature. The earliest review was published in 1904 in the *British Medical Journal* by Pearson.[6] He presented combined data on enteric fever inoculations from data provided by the British Army in India and South Africa. Another classic paper was published by Goldberger[7] in the *Bulletin of the Hygienic Laboratory* in 1907. It combined data on transmission rates of typhoid using data in reports published from 1881 to 1906. (The Hygienic Laboratory later became the U.S. National Institutes of Health.) One of the more influential developers of systematic review methods in the social sciences was G.V. Glass, whose 1981 textbook is still used.[8] Glass was also the first to use the term "meta-analysis." Researchers in health care quickly found that the systematic review methods were useful to address unanswered clinical questions.

One of the first well-done systematic reviews in modern health care was by Linus Pauling on the usefulness of vitamin C in relation to the common cold.[9] He used research current in the 1960s as well as research from Minnesota in the late 1930s and early 1940s. After all of the data were combined, the systematic review indicated that vitamin C could likely help ward off the common cold and reduce symptoms if a cold developed, but the data are still inconclusive. Research continues sporadically. Tom Chalmers,[10] considered to be one of the founders and developers of the systematic review methodology in health care, used Pauling's systematic review as the basis of his 1975 trial on vitamin C that was funded by the U.S. National Institutes of Health—the same research to which we referred in Chapter 2: Therapy, Prevention and Control, and Quality Improvement. The trial involved patients who ascertained if they were taking vitamin C or sugar—thereby breaking the code and canceling the effects of blinding.

Other Names

Systematic reviews have historically been given many names, which is consistent with any new and developing area, especially one that develops across disciplines and continents. These various names are important for retrieval of systematic review articles, especially the reviews that were published before indexers started to recognize them as systematic reviews and provide appropriate index terms. For MEDLINE, the publication types that make retrieval of certain types of articles, including meta-analyses, much easier were introduced in 1991. Systematic review articles have been called:

- systematic review or systematic overview
- meta-analysis, metaanalysis, meta analysis, metanalysis, or met-analysis
- meta-analytic review or meta-analytic overview
- meta-synthesis, metasynthesis, meta synthesis, met-synthesis
- quantitative review or quantitative overview
- quantitative synthesis
- integrative review or integrative overview

- integrative research review or overview
- research integration or research integration overview
- collaborative review or collaborative overview
- methodologic or methodological review or overview
- meta-regression, metaregression, or mega-regression (regression is a statistical technique used to combine data and ascertain if risk or protective factors such as age or severity of illness contribute to outcomes)

Overview versus Review

The term "overview" has the connotation of being a systematic review for some people. Geography tends to dictate the definition of the 2 terms *review* and *overview*. Publications called overviews done in Europe and British Commonwealth countries tend to be systematic reviews whereas in the United States an "overview" is often a narrative (traditional) review article. For example, the study by Macharia et al [11] was done in Canada. It is definitely a systematic review that collects and synthesizes the evidence on improving patient appointment keeping. The bottom line is that the rate of appointment keeping can be increased, but it takes time and effort, and may include telephone calls, mailed individualized reminders, and contracting with the patients. In contrast, the paper by Wattenberg,[12] published in the United States, is very much a narrative review of chemoprevention, with no description of how the literature used was identified and chosen.

No current information retrieval techniques can be used to tell which category of reviews an "overview" belongs: only a reading of the methods section of each can identify if an overview is a systematic review article or a narrative review article.

WHY ARE SYSTEMATIC REVIEWS DONE?

A systematic review is done for 5 major reasons:

1. **To get to a "bottom line" using all studies on a topic.** More than 1 study may have been done on a question or a closely related question. For example, no definite conclusion has been reached about the maximum amount of time after onset of symptoms that thrombolytic therapy should be administered to patients with myocardial infarction. Systematic reviews have been done and analysis across studies shows that as soon as possible after symptoms start is the ideal time to start thrombolysis, and a natural maximum time seems to exist beyond which the treatment no longer provides benefit. The evidence seems to suggest the ideal timing may be in the range of 6 hours after symptom onset.

2. **To increase the precision of estimates** of the effects of a treatment, of etiology and causation, or of another topic. Precise estimates of the effect of an intervention often need to be calculated before a study is funded. Studies with small differences between interventions or therapies need to study substantial numbers of people and their outcomes. Projected large differences indicate that smaller numbers of people can be studied. We can also combine small studies to give us a more definitive answer and more quickly if we combine data. As an example of this, Frick et al[13] assessed the rate of myocardial infarction in men with high levels of cholesterol. Approximately 2.5% of the men in the study had a myocardial infarction during the 5-year follow-up. If we needed 250 "events," or myocardial infarctions before we could come to a precise estimate of the effect of the drug gemfibrozil, we would need to study 10,000 men. Although a study of this size is possible, it is improbable that it would be financed by routine funding agencies. As an alternative to the large study, we can use the studies on gemfibrozil already published, complete a meta-analysis of the data, and come to a more precise estimate without enrolling a single new patient.

3. **To increase our understanding of an issue that relates to patients in clinically relevant subgroups.** For example, studies of patients with heart problems may include a small proportion with diabetes mellitus. By combining data across several studies for the smaller number of patients with diabetes, researchers can more fully evaluate the effect of the comorbidities (diabetes and acute coronary syndromes). Also, the condition or disease may be sufficiently rare that it is difficult to assemble enough patients to study, even when using more than 1 clinical center or city for recruitment.

4. **To resolve discrepancies in findings.** Small studies of similar interventions in similar patients can have conflicting results. Either a larger study or a systematic review of the already-published studies may provide the definitive answer.

5. **To plan new studies.** Granting agencies often require a formal calculation of the needed numbers of patients to test a study hypothesis. A meta-analysis is becoming the standard method of doing this calculation and of providing data to substantiate the need for the study in the funding proposal and to justify the projected number of patients.

STEPS IN THE PRODUCTION OF SYSTEMATIC REVIEWS

Producing a well-done systematic review is a time- and resource-intensive process. Although some aspects of the systematic review process are still being developed, the production involves 5 specific steps. Any review article produced using and reporting these steps is considered to be a systematic review article:

1. Problem formulation
2. Identification and selection articles for inclusion
3. Data extraction for analysis
4. Analysis and statistical confirmation—production of the results
5. Presentation of results

Step 1: Problem Formulation

Problem formulation must include not only the question but also the interventions, populations, settings, outcomes, duration, and the inclusion and exclusion criteria for the individual studies. These components may vary according to the question to be addressed. The purpose or objective of the review is the foundation and sets the stage for the whole review process. Establishing the question and its components initially looks easy, but it often requires substantial work and revision. The question dictates the review process and also how the results are formatted, presented, and published.

Step 2: Identifying and Selecting Studies for Inclusion

As the systematic review methodology matures, the second step is becoming more rigorous. Some early online searches involved only 2- or 3-term search strategies (e.g., screening and colorectal neoplasia, neither of which is an index term in MEDLINE). Often, the searching process starts with a comprehensive search for narrative and systematic review articles before searching for primary studies. This is done for 2 main reasons. The first is to verify that a systematic review has not already been done on the topic. Second, the bibliographies of any narrative or systematic review can provide citations for the new systematic review or hints about search methods and strategies.

Searching for studies or documents with potential for inclusion in systematic reviews often includes some of the following techniques or processes:

- Searching multiple general and specific bibliographic (e.g., MEDLINE, EMBASE) and other databases (e.g., funding or research databases)
- Complex, multifaceted searching strategies using index terms, textwords, and other database-specific techniques and terminologies
- Citation tracking using *Science Citation Index* or *Social Sciences Citation Index,* Scopus, or Google Scholar to determine which new articles have included the relevant studies and review articles in their bibliographies (i.e., which new studies have cited this important study that I have identified?)

- Hand searches of specific journals if such topic-specific journals exist
- Hand searches of conference proceedings and meeting abstracts and other "gray literature"
- Related articles searching (e.g., in PubMed and Ovid)
- Contact with authors and other experts in the field
- Contact with professional organizations and government departments, including the U.S. Centers for Disease Control and Prevention, and other, similar, national reporting agencies
- Contact with manufacturers if you are interested in commercial interventions
- Scanning bibliographies of review articles, selected studies, book chapters, clinical practice guidelines, health technology assessments and theses and dissertations
- Internet searching using multiple search engines designed for multiple purposes such as invisible web searching (e.g., Incy Wincy)

Much discussion has occurred in the professional library literature on how best to collect all the relevant studies for combination into a systematic review. Published studies are the easiest to collect. Studies and reports available only outside commercial publishers, often called the *gray literature* are much more difficult to collect. The gray literature includes unpublished internal company research reports, conference proceedings and abstracts, preliminary works, studies done only for submission to national drug approval agencies, preliminary studies conducted in advance of a full study to check the process and procedures, and studies that have not yet been published or submitted for publication. Gray literature retrieval is important for comprehensive systematic review articles. Many online sites exist to aid in gray literature retrieval.

Researchers, journal peer reviewers, and editors, being human, prefer to publish studies that have positive results (i.e., that show a difference: the drug or other intervention is shown to be effective or confirms the hypotheses of the researchers at the start of the study). Studies with negative results (i.e., that do not show a difference: the proposed surgery is no better than the standard procedure we already use or that do not provide the expected results) have been shown to be submitted less often for publication, be submitted longer after completion of the study, be rejected more often by journal editors, and be published in less well-known or in less respected journals than studies with "positive" results. This phenomenon of "less" and in "lesser" publication for trials with negative results is called **publication bias**. If these negative (i.e., no-difference studies or ones with counter-intuitive results) trials are not pursued, systematic review of only published studies can tend to overemphasize the true direction and magnitude of the combined results.

Drug companies fund many studies of their new products. Researchers employed or funded by the companies may be encouraged not to publish negative trials. This fact may also lead to meta-analyses that do not include all possible trials, and that can, therefore, be overly optimistic. Progress has been made in this area, however, by the requirement that anyone who receives funding from a major funding agency or anyone who wishes to publish in the major health care journals must register the trial before it starts and include the registration number in any publication. This requirement will lead to fewer "lost" studies.

After potential studies are identified by computer and hand searching, each study is carefully examined to ascertain whether it fits the inclusion criteria and does not meet any of the exclusion criteria set by the reviewers. The following set of inclusion and exclusion criteria comes from a meta-analysis by Schneider and Olin [14] (they called it an "overview") on the use of hydergine for treating dementia. Their inclusion and exclusion criteria for selecting articles for analysis are listed below. Frequently, more than 1 person reviews the potential studies for inclusion and exclusion to ensure that the process is rigorous and reproducible. Consensus must be obtained across the multiple reviewers before the study is included or excluded.

Inclusion Criteria

- Hydergine was used to treat elderly patients
- Patients had possible cognitive impairment or dementia at baseline
- The study was a randomized controlled trial

Exclusion Criteria

- Treatment duration was not described
- The trial was not double-blind or placebo-controlled
- The trial was either a crossover trial without first-period data or an open trial
- Hydergine was administered intravenously
- The patient sample was inappropriate
- Outcomes were inadequately reported
- End-points were nonclinical (e.g., blood levels of the drug)
- The outcome in a certain group of patients was reported and available elsewhere

Step 3: Extraction of Data

The third step is the extraction of the data from the studies and it, too, is often done in duplicate. The data from each study are put into a tabular or database format to:

- Help the reviewer understand the range of studies included
- Assess the data for possible combination (meta-analysis)

- Provide the raw data for the statistical calculations in the next step
- Get ready for formal presentation in the final publication.

This step of data extraction is important and often difficult to complete accurately and consistently. Therefore, researchers carefully construct data extraction tables or charts along with extraction rules and hints—a user's manual. The forms and instructions are pretested and the forms modified to make them easier to use and more able to accurately provide the desired information. Data extraction is complex and the task is often done in duplicate or even triplicate with multiple checks to compare results for consistency. Reconciliation of differences can be done by the data extractors themselves or by asking a third or fourth party to arbitrate. In many systematic reviews, data are extracted from studies that have met the selection criteria for most or all of the following:

- Patient numbers and their characteristics at baseline
- Study quality (poor quality studies often seem to have "better" results than similar higher quality studies). Many checklists that can be used to score study quality exist [15,16]
- Study intervention characteristics, what was done to the participants or what was the study trying to assess, including drug, dose, duration, administration route, and so on
- Follow-up duration and numbers of people who completed the trial
- Outcomes and how these are defined, measured, and assessed and by whom—blinding assessments are included here
- Confounders or other factors that might influence the results (e.g., severity of illness)
- Adverse effects—the "bad" things that can happen to participants
- The country where the study was done and published
- The year of publication
- Funding sources

Step 4: Analysis and Statistical Confirmation

At step 4 researchers determine, using both clinical common sense and statistical computations, whether the data are *similar* enough—with respect to study participants; interventions, including doses and medications; outcome measures; and character of results—so that the data across studies can be combined mathematically and statistically. If the studies and data are similar enough, the studies are considered to have *homogeneity*, and the data are pooled and analyzed together, using special meta-analytic techniques and programs. If the individual studies show *heterogeneity*, they are not similar enough for combining, and no further statistical analysis should be done using the data from the studies. At this point, if the data can be and are combined, the systematic review article becomes a meta-analysis. **Meta-analysis** is a subcategory of systematic review articles, and therefore, although the result-ing review is called a "meta-analysis," it is also a systematic review article.

Meta-analyses can be further subdivided into 2 categories. If the data from each *study* are combined—study-level data—the resulting re-port is considered to be a meta-analysis. Alternatively, if the researchers, often called *meta-analysts*, go to the investigators of each of the original studies and collect and analyze data from *each patient in each trial*, the meta-analysis is called a *collaborative review* or an **individual patient data meta-analysis**. This distinction is important both for understanding the review production process and for retrievals.

The differences among the 3 types of systematic reviews are illustrated using data from a systematic review by Hoffman et al [17] published in the *Cochrane Library*. The authors collected trials of all antihypertensive medi-cations in patients with diabetes mellitus. Patients with diabetes have a high incidence of hypertension, and it is an extremely important risk factor for cardiovascular complications. Many trials have studied all persons with hypertension, but few have included only patients with diabetes mellitus. Instead of finding their own funding and patients, Hoffman et al collected all the large studies of antihypertension medications they could find and extracted the data pertaining to patients with diabetes from each study. The following 6 studies evaluating the long-term use of any antihyperten-sive agent to reduce high blood pressure were identified. Data on all-cause mortality rates for only patients with diabetes mellitus at baseline were ex-tracted from each study and are presented as:

1182 patients were allocated to active treatment and 1220 to placebo in the six studies. After adjustment for differences in baseline age, sex, severity of hypertension and diabetes, and duration of treat-ment, the active treatment group showed a decreased risk for all-cause mortality...

Individual patient data meta-analyses are very effective and powerful, but require long-term and financial commitments from both the persons who are completing the meta-analysis and the original investigators. The original investigators must supply the data in usable format for each pa-tient. In the United Kingdom, several large meta-analyses have been done by funding an investigator from each original trial to collaboratively com-plete the individual patient data meta-analysis. One of the best known groups of reviewers is the Collaborative Group on Hormonal Factors in Breast Cancer. They completed their study on oral contraceptives in 1997 [18] and on tamoxifen in 1998. [19] These meta-analyses are powerful, and provide valuable clinical evidence; indexers at the National Library of Medicine have not provided special indexing for effective retrieval of these individual patient data meta-analyses.

An example of a study-level data meta-analysis is an extremely comprehensive review of patient decision aids by O'Connor and colleagues.[20] These decision aids present options to a patient or family in relation to the choices they have and the probable outcomes they can expect. A well-constructed decision aid incorporates the personal values the patient places on outcomes and adverse effects and helps the patient, often in conjunction with the health professional, to make the best decision possible for the situation. The authors identified 200 decision aids and collected 131 of them. Of these, 30 have been evaluated in 34 randomized controlled trials. After data extraction from these 34 studies, the combined data showed that patient decision aids contributed to:

- Increased knowledge
- More realistic expectations
- Lower decisional conflict related to feeling informed
- Increase proportion of people active in decision making
- Reduced proportion of people who remained undecided after working with the decision aid

An example of a systematic review that is not a meta-analysis is by Van et al.[21] They looked at original studies to determine if they could predict who would benefit from treatment with antidepressants. Their findings across the studies are reported not in numbers and statistical tests, but in general terms describing the results:

> **There are some indications that younger patients respond worse to tricyclics, whereas especially women appeared to have better outcomes with modern antidepressants (selective serotonin/norepinephrine reuptake inhibitors). Marital status may be related to better outcome in the case of antidepressants and cognitive-behavioral therapy. Longer duration of depression was identified as a negative predictor, most consistently in psychotherapy. In none of the treatment modalities was recurrence a negative predictor. The relation between severity of depression and outcome appeared to be complex, precluding any straightforward inferences.**

Statistics

Many of the statistics we introduced in previous chapters are also used to describe the results of systematic review articles. Usually the statistics and numbers in systematic reviews are presented as *weighted, pooled, typical, summary estimate,* or *combined* results (e.g., weighted absolute risk reduction, pooled number needed to treat, typical odds ratio, combined sensitivity and specificity, and summary estimate of the relative risk). Weighting refers to placing more emphasis on larger studies. Pooling, typical, and summary estimates refer to combining the data at the study level to come up with 1 answer for each outcome considered.

Step 5: Presentation of the Results

Systematic review articles include data and results in several formats. The raw data—the data taken from each study or from each participant—are usually presented in table form first. These tables are often accompanied by written descriptions of the similarities and differences among the studies. The columns in the first table of the paper often give the study, its name and citation number, number of participants and possibly the mean ages and gender breakdown, a brief statement on interventions, and possibly the outcomes considered in the review. This table is a combination of words and numbers.

Next are the formal combinations of data for meta-analyses—how to pull the various findings from the individual studies together to come to a new, and hopefully better (i.e., more precise), answer. The data from the individual studies are presented in another table form, with a graphic representation of the combined data and summary statistics. These tables are called forest plots or blobograms and often have 1 row per study. These tables are also supplemented with written information.

Meta-analysis Example

This tabular and graphic presentation of the raw and combined data is hard to describe. Therefore, we present findings from a meta-analysis by Delaney et al[22] using the tables representing their meta-analysis results. The systematic review was done to measure the effects on mortality and morbidity from the use of kinetic beds to prevent nosocomial pneumonia for patients on mechanical ventilation in the intensive care unit (ICU). Patients who have mechanical ventilation in the ICU are forced to be immobile and this immobility increases the risk of developing pneumonia—the most common infectious complication in ICUs. Kinetic bed therapy involves the use of a continuously rotating or oscillating bed to reduce the respiratory complications related to immobility. Table 10-1 includes the data that were extracted from each of the 15 randomized controlled trials that Delaney et al included in their systematic review. The studies are listed in the table in order of the most recent (2004) to the oldest (1998). Each trial has its own row, and each column represents a data element taken from the studies.

Statistical testing of these data showed that the trials were likely similar enough to combine into a meta-analysis (absence of heterogeneity). In this chapter we will be concerned only with the rate of new cases of nosocomial pneumonia and mortality. Meta-analysis of the data for both outcomes in forest plots are in Table 10-1 and Figures 10-1 and 10-2.

Table 10-1.
Summary of 15 Randomized Controlled Trials of Kinetic Beds to Reduce Nosocomial Pneumonia in Adults in Intensive Care Units[22]

Study	Sample size	Nosocomial pneumonia (treatment vs control)	Mortality (treatment vs control)	Ventilated days (treatment vs control)	ICU LOS (treatment vs control)	Hospital LOS (treatment vs control)
Ahrens [17]	255	14/118 vs 45/137	41/118 vs 58/137	10.8 ± 12.2 vs 10.1 ± 10.6	13.5 ± 13.2 vs 13.6 ± 11.3	NR
Bhazed [30]	22	NR	NR	NR	10 vs 18[a]	NR
Kirschenbaum [23]	37	3/17 vs 10/20	1/17 vs 2/20	21.0 ± 9.9 vs 20.0 ± 9.4	NR	NR
Macintyre [7]	103	9/52 vs 13/51	15/52 vs 14/51	NR	NR	NR
Gietzen [30]	11	NR	NR	12.4 ± 3.8 vs 35.5 ± 31.5	17.2 ± 5.8 vs 24.3 ± 11.4	25.0 ± 10.9 vs 44.9 ± 25.9
Traver [27]	103	8/44 vs 17/59	12/44 vs 19/59	3.0 (0–28) vs 3.0 (0–24)[b]	7.0 (2–43 vs 5.0 (2–53)[b]	17.5 (3–98) vs 17.0 (3–74)[b]
Whiteman [29]	69	10/33 vs 14/36	NR	13.8 ± 11.5 vs 16.1 ± 20.6	29.8 ± 27.5 vs 32.0 ± 46.5	NR
deBloisbanc [19]	110	6/69 vs 11/51	27/69 vs 14/51	6.1 ± 7.5 vs 9.9 ± 12.9	7.8 ± 6.7 vs 10.8 ± 10.0	17.0 ± 18.3 vs 18.5 ± 13.6
Nelson [24]	100	NR	4/40 vs 10/60	6.9 ± 8.9 vs 10.9 ± 15.2	8.6 ± 11.7 vs 11.2 ± 15.4	32.9 ± 30.2 vs 32.2 ± 28.2
Shapiro [25]	30	NR	NR	NR	11.4 ± 10.4 vs 12.3 ± 10.1	25.6 ± 20.8 vs 22.6 ± 19.5
Clemmer [18]	49	NR	3/23 vs 5/26	NR	20.9 ± 16.2 vs 13.9 ± 7.5	27.1 ± 16.5 vs 19.0 ± 10.5
Fink [21]	99	7/51 vs 19/48	10/51 vs 8/48	4 (0–32) vs 7 (0–74)[b]	5 (1–32) vs 8 (2–74)[b]	20 (2–201) vs 37 (5–612)[b]
Demarest [20]	30	1/16 vs 4/14	8/16 vs 6/14	NR	15.1 vs 11.4[a]	NR
Summer [26]	86	4/43 vs 7/43	10/43 vs 11/43	NR	6.7 vs 11.6[a]	NR
Gentilello [22]	65	5/27 vs 13/38	7/27 vs 5/38	8.5 ± 5.3 vs 10 ± 8.2	16.8 ± –13.6 vs 15.0 ± 15.6	NR

[a]Data reported as mean only. [b]Date reported as median and range. ICU, intensive care unit; LOS, length of stay; NR, not reported.

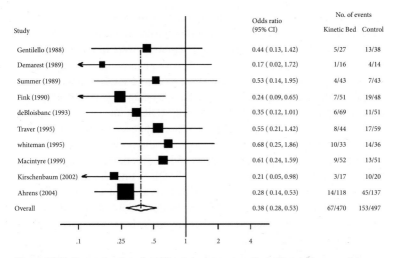

Figure 10-1. Forest plot of studies of kinetic beds to reduce the incidence of nosocomial pneumonia in adults in ICUs.[22]

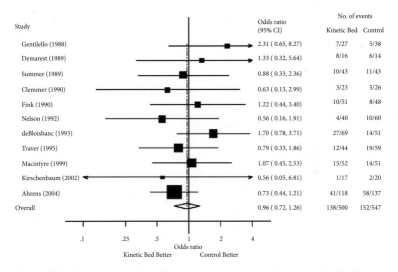

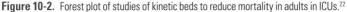

Figure 10-2. Forest plot of studies of kinetic beds to reduce mortality in adults in ICUs.[22]

Reading Forest Plots of Systematic Reviews

Looking at the forest plot for nosocomial pneumonia, we see both vertical and horizontal lines. Looking at the vertical lines, we see 2, 1 dashed and 1 solid. The *x*-axis (horizontal line) is the odds ratio (OR) line centered at 1.0. The solid horizontal line is at the OR of 1.0. Thinking back to the chapter on causation (Chapter 4), recall that the OR is a ratio for those who have the outcomes (pneumonia) or no outcomes (no pneumonia) in relation to having had the exposure (kinetic beds) or no exposure (no beds). When the OR is less than 1.0, the people who have pneumonia were in kinetic beds less often. If the OR is greater than 1, people with pneumonia were more likely to have been in kinetic beds. The vertical solid line at OR = 1 is in place to show the "dividing line" between pneumonia being associated with people in kinetic beds more (OR >1.0) or less often (OR <1.0).

Along with the OR we also have 95% confidence intervals (CIs). The CIs tell us the range of the data (i.e., its variability) if we were to repeat the study 100 times. Using statistical tests and tradition, we can say that if an OR and its 95% CI do not cross or touch the OR = 1 line for any of the studies, then we are confident that the kinetic beds are protective for pneumonia if the OR and its CIs are all <1.0. If the OR and its CIs are all >1.0, we can say with statistical confidence that kinetic beds are associated with an increased rate of pneumonia.

The forest plot has 11 horizontal lines above the x-axis. The top 10 represent 1 study (or study group) per line. The 11th line is a summary obtained by analyzing the data from all 10 trials together to come to 1 final answer. The solid line for each study represents the spread of the CI for each study. Each of the trial lines has a central box of varying size. The box's position in relation to the OR is the "best" estimate of the OR. The size of the box is a relative representation of the size of the trial—the larger the box, the more people and events that trial represents. You can check this by looking at the numbers that represent each trial to the right of each trial's line. Note also that you can see from the numbers how many patients were in each study in each group and how many developed pneumonia.

The 11th line does not have a box but has instead an open diamond. This change of symbols is a visual trigger to indicate a summary of the single trials listed above. The width of the diamond represents its CIs. The horizontal dashed line shows the summary estimate of the OR and goes through the middle of the diamond. We can see that the summary OR is quite a distance from the OR = 1.0 line. The summary estimate of the effect of kinetic beds is at the OR = 0.38. This OR is considerably less than 1.0. We can then assume from this representation of the studies and their summary that the kinetic beds are strongly associated with a substantial reduction in the incidence of pneumonia for ventilated patients in the ICU. This reduction can be said to be a statistically significant reduction in the incidence of pneumonia in patients in the ICU with mechanical ventilation and who are given kinetic beds.

Looking at the individual trial lines (and their numbers), we see that some of them have CIs that "cross" 1.0; 7 trials have crossing CIs to be exact. Three trials have ORs and CIs that do not cross 1.0. This means that 7 of the 10 trials did not show a statistically significant reduction in nosocomial pneumonia for mechanically ventilated patients and 3 trials did show a reduction. Putting the data for the 10 trials together we came to 1 bottom line—kinetic beds do reduce pneumonia by 62% in the ICU in those patients who are mechanically ventilated.

Next we move to the issue of a reduction in mortality in the same studies and patients. Review the forest plot in Figure 10-2 and see if you can answer the following questions. The answers follow.

1. How many studies are in this forest plot?
2. How many patients are in each group for the summary estimation?
3. How many of them died in each group for the summary estimation?
4. How many of the individual studies showed a statistically significant reduction in mortality with kinetic beds?
5. How many of the individual studies showed a statistically significant increase in mortality with kinetic beds?
6. Does the meta-analysis (summary estimate) show any increases? Decreases? in mortality?

The mortality data are very different from the data on nosocomial pneumonia. Answering the questions above:

1. We are now dealing with 11 studies instead of 10.
2. 138 of the 500 patients in the kinetic beds died and 152 of the 547 patients in the nonkinetic beds died. The **differences** in the rates of mortality are not all that large between the 2 groups.
3. See answer 2.
4. No studies showed a statistically significant reduction in mortality.
5. No studies showed a statistically significant increase in mortality.
6. The summary estimate of the OR for mortality is 0.96—quite close to 1.0. The 95% CI ranges from 0.72 to 1.26 and it certainly crosses 1.0.

Therefore we can say that although the kinetic beds contributed to less nosocomial pneumonia, this difference did not translate over to a difference in mortality.

SUMMARY

Systematic reviews and meta-analyses tend to be prepared more carefully and concentrate more on collection and presentation of evidence than other review articles. DiCenso and colleagues[23] list the features of systematic reviews in order of their clinical importance to a topic in their textbook on evidence-based nursing. They include:

- A focus that addresses a sensible clinical question
- Strong retrieval methods that suggest that important, relevant studies were not missed
- Primary studies to be included are of high methodological quality

- Checks made that assessments of studies were reproducible
- Studies and their results were similar and shown to be similar if results were combined using meta-analytic techniques

Knowing how to read and complete systematic reviews are important skills for librarians and clinicians to develop. Librarians have played a vital role in carrying out many systematic reviews in health care and in those organizations such as the Cochrane Collaboration and Campbell Collaboration who value and produce systematic reviews. The discipline of librarianship is also ripe for summaries of our professional knowledge base. Although we lack the levels of evidence such as many randomized controlled trials, many other kinds of evidence can be combined into intelligent summaries. *Library Trends* has produced an issue on research methods for librarians and two papers are on systematic reviews and meta-analyses.[24,25] To learn how to do systematic reviews in health sciences, the best teaching tool is likely the *Cochrane Handbook for Systematic Reviews of Interventions*.[26]

SEARCHING METHODOLOGY

Sources of Systematic Reviews

Systematic reviews and meta-analyses reside in all databases. Retrieval ease varies. Several sources that include only systematic reviews exist. Those interested in reviews can use any of the following:

- DARE is the Database for Abstracts of Reviews of Effects. It is a large, free source of abstracts and summaries of health-related systematic reviews from York University, Centre for Reviews and Dissemination in the United Kingdom (http://www.crd.york.ac.uk/crdweb/).
- Cochrane Collaboration is a worldwide group of volunteers who maintain a database of randomized controlled trials and then provide these trials to systematic reviewers. Many ways exist to access the Cochrane Reviews, including some countries with unlimited access. Everyone has access to the abstracts of the reviews (http://www.cochrane.org/reviews/).
- Campbell Collaboration is similar to the Cochrane Collaboration except that they cover crime and justice, education, and social welfare (http://www.campbellcollaboration.org/index.asp).
- Health-Evidence.ca is an example of a specialized, online database that includes reviews of public health information for decision makers (http://health-evidence.ca/). They include 2-page summaries of reviews, something that public health administrators value in their quest for evidence on which to base policy decisions.

MEDLINE

The three types of systematic review articles, systematic reviews, meta-analyses of individual studies, and meta-analyses of individual patient data, each requires its own retrieval process in MEDLINE. To the MEDLINE indexers, a review article summarizes existing literature while a meta-analysis produces new information—quite a different approach to understanding reviews from the one we have presented. In MEDLINE systematic reviews that are not meta-analyses are indexed using the publication type REVIEW. To distinguish it from other nonsystematic review articles, the textwords MEDLINE, CINAHL, handsearch, and so on can be used as textwords ANDed in with the REVIEW (publication type). Indexers also index for the study type used in the meta-analysis—e.g., a systematic review article on a therapy topic will be indexed using clinical trials as topic (MeSH) or randomized controlled trials as topic (MeSH), whereas a diagnostic systematic review article would be indexed with sensitivity and specificity (MeSH); an etiology systematic review article would be indexed with case-control studies (MeSH), cohort studies (MeSH) or risk (MeSH); and a prognosis systematic review article would be indexed with cohort studies (MeSH). Meta-analyses have both a MeSH and publication type to use in retrievals along with appropriate textwords—meta-analysis (publication type) or meta-analysis as topic (MeSH) or meta-analysis (textword). Indexing for individual patient data meta-analyses has not been formalized, and retrieval is difficult, because most of these meta-analyses are indexed as original studies.

MeSH, Subheadings, Publication Types, and Textwords

The following terms (or any term) can be ANDed with review.pt. to increase the probability of getting systematic reviews and meta-analysis as retrievals.

Electronic or bibliographic database:
MEDLINE* (note MEDLINE as a textword retrieves review articles in which a MEDLINE search has been run to retrieve the articles for inclusion)
HSTAT or Medlars* or GratefulMed or PubMed* or Healthstar
CINAHL
Psychinfo* or psycinfo* or psychlit* or psyclit* (make sure you use both correct and incorrect spellings)
Embase* or Excerpta medica
Scisearch or Science Citation Index or isi or citation database: or web of science
Ovid or EBSCO or Winspirs or Blaise or BIDS or LILACS or BLAISE or Silverplatter or Sports discus or ERIC etc.

MeSH (Medical Subject Headings — Index Terms)

Databases (can be exploded)*
Medline*
Meta analysis as topic*

Clinical protocols
Clinical trials as topic (can be exploded)
Clinical trials, phase i as topic
Clinical trials, phase ii as topic
Clinical trials, phase iii as topic
Clinical trials, phase iv as topic
Cohort studies (can be exploded)
Consensus development conferences as topic (can be exploded)
Consensus development conferences, NIH as topic
Controlled clinical trials as topic (can be exploded)
Databases, bibliographic
Follow-up studies
Guidelines as topic
Longitudinal studies (can be exploded)
Medlars (can be exploded)
Odds ratio
Practice guidelines as topic
Prospective studies
Randomized controlled trials as topic
Review literature as topic (can be exploded)

Subheadings

Diagnostic use* (can be exploded)

Publication Types

Meta-analysis*
Review*

Guideline
Practice guideline
Review academic
Review literature
Review multicase
Review of reported cases
Review tutorial
Scientific integrity review
Technical report

---

*Indicates a preferred term as determined in the Clinical Hedges Study.[27]

Twin study
Validation studies

Textwords (Same List Is Used for All 4 Databases)

Associated*
Control:*
Effectiveness*
Meta-analys*
Meta-analysis*
Risk:*
Search:*
Systematic review:*

Bibliographic search:
Clinical trial:
Cochrane
Cohort stud:
Cohort:
Collaboration:
Collaborative overview:
Collaborative review:
Collaborative stud:
Computer search:
Computerized database:
Computerised database:
Computerized literature search:
Computerised literature search:
Consensus:
Control event rate
CER
Critically appraise:
Data extraction:
Data synthesis:
Database:
Database search:
Der simonian
Dersimonian
Effect size:
Electronic database:
Exclusion criteri:
Experimental event rate:
EER

---

*Indicates a preferred term as determined in the Clinical Hedges Study.[27-30]

Fixed effect:
Fixed effect model:
Fixed effects model:
Gray literature
Grey literature
Handsearch:
Hand search:
Hazard ratio:
Hazards ratio:
HR
Heterogen:
Homogen:
Inclusion criteri:
Individual patient data:
Integrative overview:
Integrative research review:
Integrative research overview:
Integrative review:
Literature review:
Literature search:
Management plan:
Management review:
Mantel haenszel
Manual search:
Medical literature:
Meta-analytic overview:
Meta-analytic review:
Meta-regression:
Meta-synthes:
Metaanalys:
Metanalys:
Metaregression:
Methodologic overview:
Methodologic review:
Methodological overview:
Methodological review:
Number needed to treat
NNT
Number needed to harm
NNH
Odds ratio
OR
Online search:
Overview:

Peto
Peto odds ratio
Peto OR
Pool:
Pooled data:
Prospective cohort:
Prospective stud:
Published article:
Published literature:
Published source:
Quantitative overview:
Quantitative review:
Quantitative synthesis:
Random effect:
Random effect model:
Random effects model:
Randomized clinical trial:
Randomised clinical trial:
Randomized controlled trial:
Randomised controlled trial:
Randomized trial:
Randomised trial:
Reference standard:
Relative risk
RR
Relative risk reduction
RRR
Relative risk increase
RRI
Relative benefit increase
RBI
Relative benefit reduction
RBR
Relevant article:
Research integration:
Research overview:
Research review:
Risk difference
RD
Search strateg:
Search term:
Selection criteri:
Source:
Standardized mean difference

Standardised mean difference
SMD
Summarize studies
Summarize data
Summarise studies
Summarise data
Survey:
Systematic overview:
Systematic review:
Weighted event rate:
Weighted mean difference
WMD

CINAHL (CUMULATIVE INDEX TO NURSING AND ALLIED HEALTH LITERATURE)

Index Terms, Subheadings, and Publication Types

Index Terms

Confidence intervals*

"Abstracting and indexing" (can be exploded)
Biofeedback
CINAHL database
Clinical trials (can be exploded)
Cochrane library
Collaboration
Computerized literature searching (can be exploded)
Computerized literature searching, end user
Databases (can be exploded)
EMBASE
Epidemiological research
ERIC database
Full text databases, health
Health sciences indexes (can be exploded)
Integrative medicine
Literature review (can be exploded)
Literature searching (can be exploded)
Mantel-Haenszel test
Medical literature
Medlars (can be exploded)
MEDLINE

---

*Indicates a preferred term as determined in the Clinical Hedges Study.[28]

Meta analysis
Occupational therapy systematic evaluation of evidence
Odds ratio
Physiotherapy databse
Practice guidelines
Prospective studies (can be exploded)
Protocols (can be exploded)
Psycinfo
PubMed
Quantitative studies
Reference databases (can be exploded)
Reference databases, health (can be exploded)
Research methodology (can be exploded)
Resource databases, health (can be exploded)
Search engines
SportsDiscus
Surveys (can be exploded)
Systematic review
Toxlit
Treatment outcomes (can be exploded)
Twins
Validation studies

Subheadings

Drug therapy*

Publication Types

Review*
Systematic review*

Critical path
Nursing interventions
Practice guidelines
Protocol

EMBASE

Index Terms, Subheadings, and Publication Types

Index Terms

Methodology* (can be exploded)

---

*Indicates a preferred term as determined in the Clinical Hedges Study.[30]

CINAHL
Clinical protocol
Clinical study (can be exploded)
Clinical trial (can be exploded)
Cohort analysis
Controlled study (can be exploded)
Database
Dersimonian methods
EMBASE
ERIC
Fixed effects analysis
Fixed effects methods of mantel haenszel
Fixed effects model
Follow up
Literature review
Literature
Longitudinal study
Medical information
Medical literature
MEDLINE
Meta analysis
Meta regression analysis
Meta-analysis
Metasynthesis research
Organization (can be exploded)
Phase 1 clinical trial
Phase 2 clinical trial
Phase 3 clinical trial
Phase 4 clinical trial
Pooled analysis
Pooled data analysis
Practice guideline (can be exploded)
Prospective study
PsycINFO
Random effects
Random effects methods
Random effects model
Random effects of dersimonian and laird
Randomized controlled trials
Regression analysis
Review
Scientific literature (can be exploded)
Systematic review
Web of science

Subheadings

None

Publication Types

Review*

PsycINFO

Index Terms, Subheadings, and Publication Types

Index Terms

Treatment** (can be exploded)

Automated information retrieval (can be exploded)
Cohort analysis
Computer searching
Databases
Electronic communication
Followup studies
Information services
Information systems (can be exploded)
Literature review
Longitudinal studies (can be exploded)
Management planning
Meta-analysis
Prospective studies
Treatment guidelines

Subheadings

Research review

Publication Types

Clinical trial
Followup studies
Literature review
Longitudinal study
Meta-analysis
Prospective study
Research review
Treatment outcome study

---

*Indicates a preferred term as determined in the Clinical Hedges Study.[30]
**Indicates a preferred term as determined in the Clinical Hedges Study.[28]

INDEXING EXAMPLES

We have included several examples because the indexing can be complicated across the databases. Indexing is shown in Ovid syntax.

Indexing Example 1: Non Meta-analysis Systematic Review

van Sleuwen BE, Engelberts AC, Boere-Boonekamp MM, Kuis W, Schulpen TW, L'Hoir MP. Swaddling: a systematic review. *Pediatrics.* 2007 Oct;120(4):e1097-1106.

Textwords (in the Title and Abstract of the Article)

Systematic review
Systematically reviewing
MEDLINE indexing
Review.pt.

MEDLINE INDEXING

Review.pt.

CINAHL INDEXING

Cochrane library.sh.
Psycinfo.sh.
Pubmed.sh.
Systematic review.pt.

EMBASE INDEXING

Review.sh.
Systematic review.sh.
Review.pt.

Indexing Example 2: Meta-analysis of Randomized Controlled Trials

Scott-Sheldon KA, Kalichman SC, Carey MP, Fielder RL. Stress management interventions for HIV+ adults: A meta-analysis of randomized controlled trials. *Health Psychol.* 2008;27;(2):129-139.

Textwords (in the Title and Abstract of the Article)

Meta-analysis
Randomized controlled trial
Meta-analysis

Meta-analytic review
Randomized controlled trials

MEDLINE INDEXING

Randomized controlled trials as topic.sh.
Meta-analysis.pt.

CINAHL INDEXING

ERIC database.sh.
Meta-analysis.sh.
Systematic review.pt.

EMBASE INDEXING

Controlled clinical trial.sh.
Clinical trial.sh.
meta-analysis.sh.
Systematic review.sh.

Indexing Example 3: Meta-synthesis of Qualitative Research

Noyes J, Popay J. Directly observed therapy and tuberculosis: How can a systematic review of qualitative research contribute to improving services: A qualitative meta-synthesis. *J Adv Nurs.* 2007;57(3):227-243.

Textwords (in the Title and Abstract of the Article)

Systematic review
Qualitative meta-synthesis
Qualitative systematic review
Synthesize data

MEDLINE INDEXING

Qualitative research.sh.
Meta-analysis.pt.
Review.pt.

CINAHL INDEXING

CINAHL database.sh.
Clinical trials.sh.

Cochrane Library.sh.
Embse.sh.
Medline.sh.
Meta-analysis.sh.
Psycinfo.sh.
Pubmed.sh.
Qualitative studie.sh.
Systematic review.sh.
Systematic review.pt.

Indexing Example 4: Meta-analysis of Meta-analyses

Grissom, RJ. The magical number 7 +/– 2: Meta-meta-analysis of the probability of superior outcome in comparisons involving therapy, placebo, and control. *Consult Clin Psychol.* 1996;64(5):973-982.

Textwords (in the Title and Abstract of the Article)

Meta-analysis
Meta-analytics

MEDLINE INDEXING

Meta-analysis.pt.

CINHAL INDEXING

Not indexed.

EMBASE INDEXING

Meta-analysis.sh.

PSYCINFO INDEXING

Not indexed.

PROVEN STRATEGIES

Many filters exist for retrieving systematic reviews, meta-analyses, and individual patient meta-analyses across many databases and search interfaces (http://www.york.ac.uk/inst/crd/intertasc/sr.htm). The filters developed by the authors of this text are the following table.

Search Strategies (Filters) Derived during the Clinical Hedges Study[27-30]

Filter*	MEDLINE	CINAHL†	EMBASE	PsycINFO
Sensitive	search:.tw. OR meta analysis. mp,pt. OR review.pt. OR di.xs. OR associated.tw.	meta analy:.mp. OR review.pt. OR systematic review.pt.	exp methodology OR search:.tw. OR review.pt.	risk:.tw. OR search:.tw. OR exp treatment
Specific	MEDLINE.tw. OR systematic review.tw. OR meta analysis. pt.	meta analys:.tw. OR systematic review.tw.	meta-analysis.tw. OR systematic review.tw.	meta-analysis.tw. OR search:.tw.
Minimize difference between Sensitivity and Specificity	meta analysis. mp,pt. OR review.pt. OR search:.tw.	confidence intervals.sh. OR dt.fs. OR review.pt.	meta-analys:.mp. OR search:.tw. OR review.pt.	control:.tw. OR effective-ness.tw. OR risk:.tw.

*See the Introduction for a description of how to use these filters and where to find them in Ovid and PubMed.

† In 2009 CINAHL will only be offered through EBSCO. The CINAHL search strategies have been translated and are available for use in EBSCO.

EXERCISES

Note that the search possibilities (answers) are detailed in the Appendix. Obesity is a complex topic and much has been written on the topic. Because of the complexities, multiple interest groups, and large literature, systematic reviews can play a major role in understanding obesity and its research and getting this knowledge out into the community and applied.

1. Does obesity in adults cause depression? This is complex to search because searching cannot easily differentiate between depression causing obesity or obesity causing depression. Try to limit your retrievals to those studies in which the obesity came first and caused the depression.

2. Sugar-sweetened beverages, and lots of them, have had a place in the lives of many adolescents. Is the consumption of sugar-sweetened beverages associated with obesity in adolescents or children?

REFERENCES

1. French JA, Pedley TA. Clinical practice. Initial management of epilepsy. *N Engl J Med.* 2008;359:166-176.

2: Heard KJ. Acetylcysteine for acetaminophen poisoning. *N Engl J Med.* 2008;359:285-292.

3: Shoback D. Clinical practice. Hypoparathyroidism. *N Engl J Med.* 2008;359:391-403.

4. Jepson RG, Craig JC. Cranberries for preventing urinary tract infections. Update of: Cochrane Database Syst Rev. 2004;(2):CD001321. *Cochrane Database Syst Rev.* 2008;:CD001321.

5. van Sleuwen BE, Engelberts AC, Boere-Boonekamp MM, et al. Swaddling: a systematic review. *Pediatrics.* 2007;120:e1097-106.

6. Pearson K. Report on certain enteric fever inoculation statistics. *Br Med J.* 1904;3:1243-1246.

7. Goldberger J. Typhoid bacillus carriers. *Bull Hyg Lab.* 1907;35:165-174.

8. Glass GV, McGaw B, Smith ML. *Meta-analysis in Social Research.* Beverly Hills, CA: Sage Publications; 1981.

9. Pauling L. The significance of evidence about ascorbic acid and the common cold. *Proc Natl Acad Sci U S A.* 1971;68:2678-2681.

10. Macharia WM, Leon G, Rowe BH, et al. An overview of interventions to improve compliance with appointment keeping for medical services. *JAMA.* 1992;267:1813-1817.

11. Chalmers TC. Effects of ascorbic acid on the common cold. An evaluation of the evidence. *Am J Med.* 1975;58:532-536.

12. Wattenberg LW. An overview of chemoprevention: current status and future prospects. *Proc Soc Exp Biol Med.* 1997;216:133-141.

13. Frick MH, Elo O, Haapa K, et al. Helsinki Heart Study: primary prevention trial with gemfibrozil in middle-aged men with dyslipidemia. Safety of treatment, changes in risk factors, and incidence of coronary heart disease. *N Engl J Med.*1987;317:1237-1245.

14. Schneider LS, Olin JT. Overview of clinical trials of hydergine in dementia. *Arch Neurol.* 1994; 51:787-798.

15. Moher D, Jadad AR, Nichol G, er al. Assessing the quality of randomized controlled trials: an annotated bibliography of scales and checklists. *Control Clin Trials.* 1995 Feb;16:62-73.

16. Olivo SA, Macedo LG, Gadotti IC, et al. Scales to assess the quality of randomized controlled trials: a systematic review. *Phys Ther.* 2008;88:156-175.

17. Hofmann MA, Amiral J, Kohl B, et al. Hyperchomocyst(e)inemia and endothelial dysfunction in IDDM. *Diabetes Care.*1997;20:1880-1886.

18. Breast cancer and hormone replacement therapy: collaborative reanalysis of data from 51 epidemiological studies of 52,705 women with breast cancer and 108,411 women without breast cancer. *Lancet.* 1997;350:1047-1059.

19. Tamoxifen for early breast cancer: an overview of the randomised trials. Early Breast Cancer Trialists' Collaborative Group. Lancet. 1998;351:1451-1467.

20. O'Connor AM, Stacey D, Entwistle V, et al. Decision aids for people for facing health treatment or screening decisions (Review). *Cochrane Review.* 2003: CD001431.

21. Van HL, Schoevers RA, Dekker J. Predicting the outcome of antidepressants and psychotherapy for depression: a qualitative, systematic review. *Harv Rev Psychiatry.* 2008;16:225-234.

22. Delaney A, Gray H, Laupland KB, Zuege DJ. Kinetic bed therapy to prevent nosocomial pneumonia in mechanically ventilated patients: a systematic review and meta-analysis. *Crit Care.* 2006;10:R70.

23. DiCenso A, Guyatt G, Ciliska D. Evidence Based Nursing: *A Guide to Clinical Practice.* Philadelphia, PA: Elsevier Mosby; 2005.

24. Saxton M. Meta-analysis in library and information science: Method, history, and methods for reporting research. Library Trends. 2006;55:158-170.

25. McKibbon KA. Systematic reviews and librarians. *Library Trends.* 2006;55:202-215.

26. Cochrane Collaboration. *Cochrane Handbook for Systematic Reviews of Interventions.* Higgins JPT, Green S (eds). Version 5.0.0. February 2008. Accessed August 1, 2008; http://www.cochrane-handbook.org/

27. Montori VM, Wilczynski NL, Morgan D, Haynes RB for the Hedges Team. Optimal search strategies for retrieving systematic reviews from MEDLINE: analytical survey. *BMJ.* 2005;330:68. http://bmj.bmjjournals.com/cgi/reprint/330/7482/68.

28. Wong SS, Wilczynski NL, Haynes RB. Optimal CINAHL search strategies for identifying therapy studies and review articles. *J Nurs Scholarsh.* 2006;38:194-199.

29. Wilczynski NL, Haynes RB, Hedges Team. EMBASE search strategies achieved high sensitivity and specificity for retrieving methodologically sound systematic reviews. *J Clin Epidemiol.* 2007;60:29-33.

30. Eady AM, Wilczynski NL, Haynes RB. PsycINFO search strategies identified methodologically sound therapy studies and review articles for use by clinicians and researchers. *J Clin Epidemiol.* 2008;61:34-40.

11

Secondary Publications: Clinical Practice Guidelines

Ann McKibbon

Practice guidelines are "systematically developed statements to assist practitioner and patient decisions about appropriate health care for specific clinical circumstances."[1] This definition was adopted by the U.S. Institute of Medicine Committee to Advise the Public Health Service on Practice Guidelines. Guidelines are developed based on cumulated evidence and are meant to direct practice so that patients can have the care they should have and, at the same time, not be given what they do not need. Guidelines are designed for individuals or groups of practitioners. Associations, foundations, or other clinical groups produce them through committees and task forces composed of people with diverse experiences and expertise. By virtue of the sponsoring agency's backing, the developers make recommendations that can be taken as standards of care by individuals. The producers or the sponsoring agency may also disseminate the resulting guideline and its recommendations to group members for their use or to agencies for formal implementation.

Guidelines range in size and scope. A smaller guideline may be in the from of a "care map" developed by the staff of a single hospital intensive care unit to help guide and guarantee continuity of care for patients with acute stroke during their first week in the hospital. A much larger, broadly based guideline on topics such as incontinence or pressure sores may be developed for national or regional distribution and implementation. Estimates of the number of guidelines vary. In the United States, national estimates range from 1,600[2] to more than 26,000.[3] These estimates were made in the mid to late 1990s; few people try to estimate the number of guidelines available today.

CLINICAL EXAMPLE

The example for this chapter centers on universal screening of all newborn babies to identify hearing problems. Some estimates show that approximately 1 in 1000 infants have substantial hearing deficits that can be identified early and treated.[4] Of the children identified as having hearing deficits, only approximately half of these have risk factors. This means that to identify most infants with hearing deficits, screening must be universal. Thirty-nine U.S. states have implemented a screening program for all infants before 1 month of age. Because some infants in these states were not being screened as well as the infants in other states, Dr. Ned Cologne and 14 peers (physicians, nurses, and epidemiologists) were charged with updating a set of national guidelines produced in 2000.[5] To help this panel of experts in their task, the U.S. Agency for Health Care Research and Quality (AHRQ) summarized existing evidence on identification of hearing deficits in infants. The evidence was in the form of a large systematic review published as a lengthy document. A summary of their evidence and their only recommendation was published as a journal article in *Pediatrics* in July 2008.[6] The only recommendation is:

The United States Preventive Services Task Force (USPSTF) recommends screening for hearing loss in all newborn infants.

This recommendation is graded "B" which means that the committee found at least fair evidence that screening infants for hearing loss within 1 month of birth provides measurable overall benefit that outweighs costs and risks. This recommendation is identical to the recommendations in the first guideline on hearing deficits published in 2000.

METHODOLOGICAL ISSUES

Guidelines are promoted as a means for improving the quality of health care, optimizing patient outcomes, discouraging the use of ineffective or harmful interventions, improving and enabling the consistency of care, identifying gaps in evidence, and helping balance costs and outcomes through considered assessment of competing interests. Medical organizations, health services researchers, sponsors of health benefit plans, and public officials have expressed interest in their development and implementation. With this increased attention have come concerns about guidelines from individuals and groups.

Guidelines have several challenges. First, they do not take into account individual situations or clinicians or the various settings in which they can be applied. Guidelines seem to be most effective when used as general guides to specific situations. They have been used in legal situations and by health organizations to both provide and deny care to people with health care problems. Guidelines are also often out of date because of changing health care and the time it take to produce and implement the guidelines.

Depending on the subject, they may be out of date even at the time of publication. Despite these problems, more guidelines are being produced in many countries.

Opinions are strong, both for and against guidelines. For example, a Canadian survey of physician knowledge, attitudes, and use of guidelines recorded this comment from a concerned physician[7]: "Guidelines are developed simply to control costs. They should be banned in perpetuity and those who promote them should be banished to the deepest pits of hell." Not everyone feels that strongly, but almost everyone involved with health care has some feelings about the use and place of guidelines.

To address some of these concerns, questions have been raised on standardization and perfection of the specific methods used to develop guidelines; their clinical and methodological reliability; their validity; whether clinicians will interpret and apply them consistently under similar clinical circumstances; and whether, if applied properly, the guidelines will lead to the predicted health outcomes, consistency, and projected costs. To answer these questions, several groups are in the process of bringing order and quality to development of guidelines and evaluating their impact. The Canadian Task Force on the Periodic Health Examination and the U.S. Preventive Services Task Force (USPSTF) are national organizations of health care professionals who developed large collections of well-done, evidence-based guidelines for their respective countries in the 1990s. The USPSTF has continued their work and their website includes over 100 guidelines (http://www.ahrq.gov/clinic/uspstf/uspstopics.htm). The websites provide comprehensive assistance for primary health care practitioners and others who deal with routine preventive care. The Canadian and U.S. organizations have worked together and shared expertise and evidence resources; the resulting guidelines, although similar, reflect national and regional differences. In addition, the U.S. Congress has assigned AHRQ responsibility for determining the definitions and attributes of practice guidelines and their evaluation.[8]

EVIDENCE-BASED PRACTICE CENTERS

The AHRQ has designated 14 evidence-based practice centers to assemble evidence that will provide the basis for production of clinical practice guidelines[9]; 11 centers are located in the United States and 3 in Canada. Under contract, each center works with organizations that have requested AHRQ to produce a specific set of evidence in a report that will support guideline production. For example, McMaster University worked with the American Academy of Pediatricians and the American Psychiatric Association to produce a summary of the evidence on the diagnosis and treatment of attention deficit hyperactivity disorder in children and adults. This evidence formed the basis of several guidelines.[10,11] Each center was assigned their first topic in late 1997. Although some centers have changed over the years, many are still the same. Approximately 30 projects are ongoing at any one time. Contract costs for each evidence summary are often in the range of $250,000 per project and most take 12 months to complete.

Steps in the Production of a Clinical Practice Guideline

Guideline production usually involves a 6-step process. Some of these steps are similar to those used to produce systematic reviews. Both systematic reviews and clinical practice guidelines are summaries of published evidence—guidelines go 1 step further by providing recommended actions for clinicians, organizations, or both to ensure appropriate and cost-effective care. Before production starts, the team who will produce the guideline must be set. Resource issues and timelines are other important considerations that must be established early in the process. The 6-step process follows:

1. **Definition of the topic or process to be assessed.** This includes defining the target condition, interventions, patient population, clinical settings to be included, type of scientific evidence to be considered, and outcome measures to assess effectiveness and safety. A question is set that will direct the rest of the production process.

2. **Assessment of clinical benefits and harms** including review of scientific evidence: literature searching and retrieval based on parameters from topic definition, evaluation of individual studies, including grading of the quality of the evidence and abstraction of the results, and synthesis (ie, summary) of the evidence. Consideration of expert opinion and existing care standards are also included at this step.

3. **Consideration of resource and feasibility issues**. All care has costs, benefits, and risks, and guidelines can help plan how best to utilize existing health professionals and spend scare health care resources.

4. **Development of recommendations**, including an assessment of the strength of the recommendations and the extent to which they are supported by scientific evidence.

5. **Writing the preliminary version of the guideline** after consensus has been achieved in the team.

6. **External review of the evidence and recommendations**. This involves consideration of the clinical implications and adoption by the relevant health care community. This step often includes redrafting the recommendations and report based on input from external individual and group reviewers.

Evidence-based guidelines are based on levels of evidence: the stronger the evidence, the more faith a reader or implementer can put in the recommendation of the guideline. Recommendations are the "meat" of any guideline. They should be precise statements of specific actions to be taken or not taken in specific circumstances, and reflect the evidential strength for making that statement. For example, the Royal College of Obstetricians and Gynaecologists[12] in the United Kingdom states: "Women with multiple pregnancies are at increased risk of pre-eclampsia and should receive specialist antenatal care (Grade A)."

Heffner[13] discusses further how EBHC helps with the development of clinical practice guidelines. Although the steps in guideline development have been established since the 1980s, each group of guideline developers sets its own levels of strength of evidence. For example, the Canadian Hypertension Society Consensus Development Conference set 1 of the earliest rankings of levels of evidence, which follows.[14] Most guideline developers use a similar, but not identical, ranking of evidence.

Levels of Evidence for Rating Studies of Therapy, Prevention, and Quality Improvement

I.   A randomized controlled trial (RCT) that demonstrates a statistically significant difference in at least 1 important outcome—eg, survival or major illness; or, if the difference is not statistically significant, a RCT of adequate sample size to exclude a 25% difference in relative risk with 80% power, given the observed results.

II.   A RCT that does not meet level I criteria.

III. A nonrandomized trial with contemporaneous controls selected by some systematic method (ie, not selected by perceived suitability for 1 of the treatment options for individual patients); or subgroup analysis of a RCT.

IV.   A before and after study or case series (of at least 10 patients) with historical controls or controls drawn from other studies.

V.   Case series (at least 10 patients) without controls.

VI.   Case report (fewer than 10 patients).

Levels of Evidence for Rating Studies of Diagnosis

I.   A review that meets all of the criteria:
   (a) Independent interpretation of the test procedure (without knowledge of result of the diagnostic standard).
   (b) Independent interpretation of the diagnostic standard (without knowledge of the test procedure).
   (c) Selection of patients or subjects who are suspected, but not known, to have the disorder of interest.

(d) Reproducible description of both the test and diagnostic standard.

(e) At least 50 patients with and 50 without the disorder.

II. Meets 4 of the criteria in I.

III. Meets 3 of the criteria in I.

IV. Meets 2 of the criteria in I.

V. Meets 1 of the criteria in I.

VI. Meets none of the criteria in I.

Levels of Evidence for Rating Studies of Prognosis

I.   Inception cohort that meets these 4 criteria:
   (a) Reproducible inclusion and exclusion criteria.
   (b) Follow-up of at least 80% of subjects.
   (c) Statistical adjustment for extraneous prognostic factors (confounders).
   (d) Reproducible description of outcome measures.

II. Inception cohort, but meets only 3 of the other criteria in I.

III. Inception cohort, but meets only 3 of the other criteria in I.

IV. Inception cohort, but meets only 1 of the other criteria in I.

V. Inception cohort, but meets none of the other criteria in I.

VI. Meets none of the criteria in I.

Levels of Evidence for Rating Review Articles

I.   A review article that meets all of these criteria:
   (a) Comprehensive search for evidence.
   (b) Avoidance of bias in selection of articles.
   (c) Assessment of the validity of each cited article.
   (d) Conclusions supported by the data and analysis presented.

II. Meets only 3 of the criteria in I.

III. Meets only 2 of the criteria in I.

IV. Meets only 1 of the criteria in I.

V. Meets none of the criteria in I.

Grading System for Recommendations

Each recommendation is also given a "grade" in addition to an assessment of the level or quality of the evidence. Again, these grades differ from group to group. The grades for the Canadian Hypertension Society are as follows:

A. The recommendation is based on one or more studies at level I.

B. The best evidence was at level II.

C. The best evidence was at level III.

D. The best evidence was lower than level III, and included expert opinion.

Another set of gradings for recommendations is that used by the Canadian Task Force on the Periodic Health Examination and the U.S. Preventive Services Task Force for their recommendations. This grading is used more often than the Canadian Hypertension Society list:

A. Strong evidence to support the recommendation.
B. Weak evidence to support the recommendation.
C. No evidence to support or refute the recommendation.
D. Weak evidence to refute the recommendation.
E. Strong evidence to refute the recommendation.
I. There is insufficient evidence (in quantity, quality, or both) to make a recommendation; however, other factors may influence decision making.

Two examples of recommendations from the Canadian Task Force show these gradings and levels [15]:

1. Fair evidence exists to include colonoscopy for the periodic health examination of patients in kindreds with cancer family syndrome (III, B).
2. Insufficient evidence exists to include or exclude multiphasic screening in the periodic health examination of patients >40 years old if they have no family history of colorectal cancer (I, C).

ALTERNATIVE NAMES

The following list includes some, but not all, of the names or labels that have been used to refer to clinical guidelines. They are from a MEDLINE search strategy produced by the British Columbia Office of Health Technology Assessment Centre for Health Services and Policy Research.[17] This list can be used for retrieval in any searching system.

clinical protocol:
clinical or medical guideline:
clinical or medical standard:
clinical or medical protocol:
clinical or medical recommend:
clinical or medical statement:
clinical or medical criteri:
clinical or medical polic:
clinical or medical option:
clinical or medical intervention:
practice or practise or care guideline:
practice or practise or care standard:
practice or practise or care protocol:
practice or practise or care recommend:
practice or practise or care statement:
practice or practise or care criteri:
practice or practise or care parameter:

practice or practise or care polic:
practice or practise or care option:
practice or practise or care intervention:
position paper: or statement:
health guideline:
health planning guideline:
flowchart:
consensus development conference:
physician's practice pattern: or physicians' practice pattern:
practice or practise pattern:
medical or clinical necessity:
medical or clinical indicator:
reference standard:
treatment guideline: standard: or protocol:
treatment parameter: or polic:
treatment option: or intervention:
prefer: (practice or practise or treat:)
planning (guideline: or standard: or protocol:)
planning (recommend: or statement: or criteri:)
performance (guideline: or standard: or protocol:)
performance (recommend: or statement: or criteri:)
planning or performance parameter:
appropriate (evaluat: or care)
(guideline: or standard: or protocol:) and criteri:
(medical or clinical) review and criteri:
(practice or practice) review and criteri:
(medical or clinical) review:
(practice or practice) review:
(management or care or performance) review and criteri:
performance measure:
(clinical or critical) pathway:
care map:
algorithm:
consensus develop conference:

The ":" means truncation—it will retrieve multiple endings on search words (for example, map: will retrieve map, maps, mapping, mapped, and also maple).

STRUCTURED ABSTRACTS FOR CLINICAL PRACTICE GUIDELINES

Just as the health care community has moved to implement more informative abstracts of clinical studies, a proposed structure for abstracts of

clinical guidelines has been developed and implemented by users and producers of guidelines.[18] Structured abstracts of any body of literature have
3 important functions. (1)The structure ensures that authors provide information that is crucial to their readers. Although an abstract's purpose is
to provide information so a person can determine whether the full text of
the document is needed, many people only read the abstract before acting.
(2) The abstracts also aid with retrieval by ensuring that important concepts
like the methods or certain outcomes are included and therefore available
for searching. (3) A structured abstract for guidelines enables one to understand the processes that went into development of the guideline, if it is
important to the searching question, and to enhance retrieval. The section
headings for a structured abstract of clinical practice guidelines include:

- Objective
- Option
- Outcomes
- Evidence
- Values
- Benefits, Harms and Costs
- Recommendations
- Validation
- Sponsors

A summary of the information to be included in each section follows,
using a guideline on prevention of postoperative pain from the Society of
Gynecologists and Obstetricians of Canada as an illustrative example.[19]
Later in the chapter we will look at the heading and sections from the guideline on hearing screening for newborn infants that we used as our clinical
example at the start of the chapter [5]

Objective

The purpose of this section is to provide key information for the readers to
decide if the guideline is relevant. The Objective identifies the health problem (disease or condition) on which the guideline concentrates; the health
care strategies that will address the problem; the patients to whom the guideline applies; and the care providers who are expected to use the guideline.

**To develop a Canadian consensus document with recommendations on
maternal screening for fetal aneuploidy (e.g., Down syndrome and trisomy
18) in pregnancy.**

Options

The Options section identifies the key health care options so that the reader
can determine whether the guideline is relevant to his or her situation.

It identifies the health care options that will be examined in the guideline. Often these are just listed in this section, and will be addressed more thoroughly later under the Benefits, Harms, and Costs section.

> **The areas of clinical practice considered in formulating this guideline are prevention and prophylaxis, treatment, both medical and alternative, and patient education.**

Outcomes

The main outcomes considered in the guideline are listed. This section often includes health outcomes, often in order of importance (mortality, morbidity, signs and symptoms, health care use, health-related behaviors, and quality of life), along with the main economic outcomes, and outcomes related to health care procedures or tests.

> **Pregnancy screening for fetal aneuploidy started in the mid 1960s, using maternal age as the screening test. New developments in maternal serum and ultrasound screening have made it possible to offer all pregnant patients a non-invasive screening test to assess their risk of having a fetus with Down syndrome or trisomy 18 to determine whether invasive prenatal diagnosis tests are necessary. This document will review the options available for non-invasive screening and make recommendations for Canadian patients and health care workers.**

Evidence

The purpose of this section is to provide information on the guideline development process so that a reader can decide if he or she is confident that the collection and synthesis methods included key relevant studies. The Evidence section includes methods for collecting the evidence (search methods), search results, methods for combining and analyzing the evidence, methods for assessing the strength of evidence, and planned updates or reviews.

> **A MEDLINE search was carried out to identify papers related to this topic that were published between 1982 and 2006. Practices across Canada were surveyed. A consensus document was drafted and reviewed by committee members.**

Values

This section provides an idea of the perspective taken during guideline development and includes a list of major organizations involved, panel membership, methods or synthesizing panel member opinions or disagreements, and panel points of view and preferences.

VALUES: The quality of evidence and classification of recommendations followed discussion and consensus by the combined committees of SOGC (Genetics, Diagnostic Imaging) and CCMG (Prenatal Diagnosis).

Benefits, Harms, and Costs

This section presents evidence on the effects of the various options on the specified outcomes. It includes potential benefits of options and the magnitude for the benefits, potential harms of the options, and the magnitude of the harms, and any cost analyses.

It is often one of the longest sections of the abstract and original guideline.

These guidelines are intended to reduce the number of amniocenteses done when maternal age is the only indication. This will have the benefit of reducing the numbers of normal pregnancies lost because of complications of invasive procedures. Any screening test has an inherent false positive rate, which may result in undue anxiety. A detailed cost-benefit analysis of the implementation of this guideline has not been done, since this would require health surveillance and research and health resources not presently available; however, these factors need to be evaluated in a prospective approach by provincial and territorial initiatives.

Recommendations

This section presents the recommendations made by the guideline developers. It lists recommendations with assigned grades, evidence levels, or both. A "good" guideline will include supporting citations linked to individual recommendations. The guideline includes 11 recommendations, which in this case are not listed in the abstract but in the full text of the article. We include only the first 2 recommendations.

---

1. **All pregnant women in Canada, regardless of age, should be offered, through an informed consent process, a prenatal screening test for the most common clinically significant fetal aneuploidies in addition to a second trimester ultrasound for dating, growth, and anomalies. (I-A)**
2. **Maternal age screening is a poor minimum standard for prenatal screening for aneuploidy and should be removed as an indication**

for invasive testing. Amniocentesis/ chorionic villi sampling (CVS) should not be provided without multiple marker screening results except for women over the age of 40. Patients should be counselled accordingly. (I-A)

Note that the quality of evidence is I = randomized controlled trial evidence. The grades of evidence are the same as the Canadian Task Force on the Periodic Health Examination Care: A = "There is good evidence to recommend the clinical preventive action."

Validation

This section provides information on the involvement of outside agencies and people, what contribution they made to its development with respect to their values, and their refinement of the guideline and its developmental process. It includes a description of external peer review before publication, external pilot testing before publication, and agreement and disagreement of recommendations with those in other guidelines. Our example guideline does not have a validation section.

Sponsors

The purpose of this section is to identify the sponsoring and endorsing agencies and thus provide information on potential biases and special interests the guideline developers might have had.

Society of Gynecologists and Obstetricians of Canada.

PRESENTATION OF DATA IN GUIDELINES

Guidelines do not necessarily stick to 1 way of presenting their data. The universal hearing loss screening guideline for newborn infants includes sections on rationale, clinician considerations including options, other considerations, discussion including study findings and evidence of benefits, harms, and costs, and recommendations of the guideline and other groups.

The hearing screening guidelines used the following headings in their clinical practice guideline:

- Importance
- Benefits of detection and early treatment of hearing loss
- Harms of detection and early treatment of hearing loss
- Patient population under consideration
- Screening tests—options and accuracy
- Treatments—options and effectiveness

- Screening intervals
- Magnitude of net benefit
- Recommendation
- Recommendations of others
- Members of the Task Force who produced the guideline

SUMMARY

Clinical practice guidelines are important components of the health care literature and for patient care decision making. Although they engender feelings of both support and condemnation they are probably here to stay. The advent of electronic medical records provided the vehicle that could integrate the recommendations into direct patient care. This idea of intergration has spawned much research and development work that may soon be implemented in routine clinical and hospital care. As an example of the integration of guidelines into an electronic medical records system, Weber and colleagues[20] showed that diabetes care improved substantially when guidelines triggered care prompts to primary care physicians. Physicians were given financial incentives to follow these guidelines and meet the 9 patient goals set by the guidelines.

Di Censo and Guyatt[21] provide the most important aspects of high-quality clinical practice guidelines.

1. Are all relevant patient groups, care options, and outcomes considered?
2. Is the evidence sought and summarized carefully and appropriately?
3. Are values and preferences of involved patients and clinicians considered and considered appropriately?
4. Are all recommendations aligned and presented with their strength?

SEARCHING METHODOLOGY

Retrieval

Guidelines published in medical journals are searchable in MEDLINE and other general-purpose and specialty databases. MEDLINE uses the publication types "guideline.pt." for administrative or procedural guidelines, and "practice guideline.pt." for specific health care guidelines. CINAHL is a rich database for this material, and includes the full text of many clinical practice guidelines. Retrieval for material that is incorporated into the production of guidelines should be retrieved using terms and techniques from previous chapters. The following information is for retrieval of already produced clinical practice guidelines.

The Internet also has many good listings of clinical practice guidelines. One of the best places to start is an excellent site developed by AHRQ in conjunction with the American Medical Association and the American

Association of Health Plans (http://www.guidelines.gov/). They include many local, national, and international guidelines, provide the recommendations, and often the full text of the guideline. Several guidelines on a topic can be compared online using some of their special features. The Canadian Medical Association Infobase (http://www.cma.ca/cpgs/index.htm) lists more than 1200 clinical practice guidelines of importance to Canadians. Other nations also keep web sites of guidelines. For example the United Kingdom provides a national Library of Guidelines Specialist Library (http://www.library.nhs.uk/GuidelinesFinder/). It includes links to other national collections of guidelines (http://www.library.nhs.uk/guidelinesFinder/Page.aspx?pagename=INTER).

Haase and colleagues[22] provide searching strategies for identifying guidelines using various web tools (SUMSearch and Google Scholar). For those who wish to search for guidelines using the large bibliographic databases, searching suggestions follow. We have produced search filters for clinical practice guidelines for high-quality and all clinical practice guidelines for MEDLINE.[23]

MEDLINE Strategies for Retrieval of Clinical Practice Guidelines

Filter	MEDLINE (Ovid syntax)
High quality clinical practice guidelines*—Specific	Guideline:.tw. OR exp data collection OR recommend:.tw.
High quality clinical practice guidelines*—Sensitive	Guidelines.tw. OR practice guidelines as topic.sh OR recommend:.tw.
All clinical practice guidelines	Exp health services administration OR tu.xs (therapeutic use floating subheading) OR management.tw.

* Includes an explicit statement describing how the guideline was developed, how the evidence was identified and summarized and identified at least 1 of the participants who produced the guideline, how the guidelines recommendations were formulated, and how agreement or consensus was reached.[23]

MEDLINE

MeSH Subheadings, Publication Types, and Textwords

MeSH (Medical Subject Headings — Index Terms)

Data collection*
Health services administration* (can be exploded)

*Indicates a preferred term as determined in the Clinical Hedges Study.[23]

Practice guidelines as topic*

Consensus development conferences as topic (can be exploded)
Consensus development conferences as topic, NIH
Continuity of patient care
Cost-benefit analysis
"Costs and cost analysis" (can be exploded)
Delivery of health care (can be exploded)
"Delivery of health care (integrated)" (can be exploded)
Guideline adherence
Guidelines as topic
Health care costs
Health care costs (can be exploded)
Health care evaluation mechanisms
Health care evaluation mechanisms (can be exploded)
"Health care quality, access, and evaluation" (can be exploded)
Health care rationing
Health care reform
Health expenditures
Health planning guidelines
Health services accessibility
"Health services needs and demand" (can be exploded)
Institutional practice
Organization and administration" (can be exploded)
"Outcome and process assessment (health care)" (can be exploded)
"Outcome assessment (health care)" (can be exploded)
Physicians practice patterns
Planning techniques
Policy making
Practice management
"Process assessment (health care)"
"Quality assurance (health care)" (can be exploded)
"Quality indicators (health care)" (can be exploded)
Quality of health care (can be exploded)
Review literature as topic
Technology assessment, biomedical
Treatment outcome
Unnecessary procedures

Subheadings

Therapeutic use*
Standards

---

*Indicates a preferred term as determined in the Clinical Hedges Study.[23]

Publication Types

Consensus development conference
Consensus development conference, NIH
Guideline (can be exploded)
Practice guideline
Review literature

Textwords (Same List Is Used for All 4 Databases)

See earlier in the chapter for a list of names for clinical practice guidelines.

CINAHL (CUMULATIVE INDEX TO NURSING AND ALLIED HEALTH LITERATURE)

Index Terms, Subheadings, and Publication Types

Index Terms

Practice guidelines
Guideline adherence
Outcomes (Health Care)

Subheadings

Standards

Publication Types

Practice guidelines
Nursing interventions

EMBASE

Index Terms, Subheadings, and Publication Types

Index Terms

Practice guideline (can be exploded)
Clinical pathway
Clinical protocol
Consensus
Consensus development
Good clinical practice
Clinical practice

Outcome assessment
Outcomes research
Treatment failure
Treatment outcome

Subheadings

None

Publication Types

None

PsycINFO

Index Terms, Subheadings, and Publication Types

Index Terms

Professional standards
Professional ethics
Quality of services

Subheadings

None

Publication Types

Clinical practice guidelines
Clinical practice algorithm

EXAMPLES OF TEXTWORDS AND INDEXING USING OUR CLINICAL EXAMPLE

Citation for Our Clinical Example 1

U.S. Preventive Services Task Force. Screening for gestational diabetes mellitus: U.S. Preventive Services Task Force recommendation statement. *Ann Intern Med*. 2008 May 20;148(10):759–765.

Textwords and Index Terms Used in Our Clinical Example

Textwords (in the Title and Abstract of the Article)

Recommendation
US Preventive Services Task Force

USPSFT
Benefits and harms

MEDLINE INDEXING

Standards subheading
Practice guildline.pt.

CINAHL INDEXING

Practice guidelines
Preventive health care

EMBASE INDEXING

Practice guideline
Preventive health services

Citation for Our Clinical Example 2

Lindsay P, Bayley M, McDonald A, Graham ID, Warner G, Phillips S. Toward a more effective approach to stroke: Canadian Best Practice Recommendations for Stroke Care. *CMAJ*. 2008 May 20;178(11):1418–1425.

Textwords (in the Title and Abstract of the Article)

Best practice
Recommedation
Guideline
Consensus panel

MEDLINE INDEXING

Practice guidelines as topic.sh.
Note: did not index as practice guideline.pt.

CINAHL INDEXING

Practice guidelines.sh.

EMBASE INDEXING

Consensus.sh.
Practice guideline.sh.

Citation for Our Clinical Example 3

Steering Committee on Quality Improvement and Management, Subcommittee on Febrile Seizures. American Academy of Pediatrics.

Febrile seizures: Clinical practice guidelines for the long-term management of the child with simple seizures. *Pediatrics.* 2008 Jun;121(6):1281–1286.

Textwords (in the Title and Abstract of the Article)

Clinical practice guideline
Practice parameter

MEDLINE INDEXING

Practice guildeline.pt.

CINAHL INDEXING

Practice guidelines.sh.

PsycINFO INDEXING

Clinical practice guidelines (key concept)
Clinical practice.sh.

EXERCISES

Note that the search possibilities (answers) are detailed in the Appendix.

1. Many national and international guidelines exist that mention literacy as being important to health and wellness. Do any guidelines exist that concentrate only on literacy? If so, what countries do they represent? Try MEDLINE and any other source you can think of.

2. Go the U.S. National Guidelines Clearinghouse and find 2 guidelines that deal with palliative care for patients with heart failure. Work through the screens and "compare" these 2. See if you can discern differences in their development and if these differences have any affect on the recommendations.

REFERENCES

1. Field MJ, Lohr KN. *Clinical Practice Guidelines.* Washington, DC: National Academy Press; 1990.
2. American Medical Association. *Directory of Practice Parameters: Titles, Sources and Updates.* Chicago: American Medical Association; 1996.
3. ECRI. *Health Care Standards, 1997.* Plymouth Meeting, PA: ECRI; 1997.
4. Watkin PM. Neonatal hearing screening: have we taken the right road? Results from a 10-year targeted screen longitudinally followed up in a single district. *Audiological Med.* 2005;3:175–184.

5. U.S. Preventive Services Task Force. *Universal Screening for Hearing Loss in Newborns: U.S. Preventive Services Task Force Recommendation Statement.* AHRQ Publication No. 08–05117-EF-2, July 2008. Agency for Healthcare Research and Quality, Rockville, MD. http://www.ahrq.gov/clinic/uspstf08/newbornhear/newbhearrs.htm

6. Nelson HD, Bougatsos C, Nygren P. Universal newborn hearing screening: systematic review to update the 2001 U.S. Preventive Services Task Force Recommendation. *Pediatrics.* 2008;122:e266–e276.

7. Hayward RS, Guyatt GH, Moore KA, et al. Canadian physicians' attitudes about and preferences regarding clinical practice guidelines. *CMAJ.* 1997;156:1715–1723.

8. *Methods and Background.* U.S. Preventive Services Task Force. Agency for Healthcare Research and Quality, Rockville, MD. Accessed November 24, 2008. http://www.ahrq.gov/clinic/uspstmeth.htm.

9. Woolf SH. Do clinical practice guidelines define good medical care? The need for good science and the disclosure of uncertainty when defining "best practices." *Chest.* 1998;13:166S–1671S.

10. American Academy of Pediatrics. Subcommittee on Attention-Deficit/Hyperactivity Disorder and Committee on Quality Improvement. Clinical practice guideline: Diagnosis and evaluation of the child with attention-deficit/hyperactivity disorder. *Pediatrics.* 2000;105:1158–1170.

11. American Academy of Pediatrician. Subcommittee on Attention-Deficit/Hyperactivity Disorder and Committee on Quality Improvement. Clinical practice guideline: Treatment of the school-aged child with attention-deficit/hyperactivity disorder. *Pediatrics.* 2001;108:1033–1044.

12. UK Royal College of Obstetricians and Gynaecologists. Pre-eclampsia Study Group Statement. September, 2003. Accessed November 24, 2008. http://www.rcog.org.uk/index.asp?PageID=312.

13. Heffner JE. Does evidence-based medicine help the development of clinical practice guidelines? *Chest.* 1998;113:172S–178S. http://www.rcog.org.uk/index.asp?PageID=312; accessed August 4, 2008.

14. Carruthers SG, Larochelle P, Haynes RB, et al. Report of the Canadian Hypertension Concensus Conference: 1 Introduction. *CMAJ.* 1993;149:289–293.

15. Solomon MJ, McLeod RS. Periodic health examination, 1994 update: 2. Screening strategies for colorectal cancer. Canadian Task Force on the Periodic Health Examination. *CMAJ.*1994;150:1961–1970.

16. Audet A, Greenfield S, Field M. Medical practice guidelines: current activities and future directions. *Ann Intern Med.* 1990;113:709–714.

17. B.C. Office of Health Technology Assessment Centre for Health Services and Policy Research. *Bone Mineral Density Testing: Does the Evidence Support Its Selective Use in Well Women?* Vancouver, British Columbia; University of British Columbia; 1997; 130–131.

18. Hayward RS, Wilson MC, Tunis SR, et al. More informative abstracts of articles describing clinical practice guidelines. *Ann Intern Med.*1993;118:731–737.

19. Summers AM, Langlois S, Wyatt P, Wilson RD. Society of Obstetricians and Gynaecologists of Canada. Prenatal screening for fetal aneuploidy. *J Obstet Gynaecol Can.* 2007;29:146–179.

20. Weber V, Bloom F, Pierdon S, Wood C. Employing the electronic health record to improve diabetes care: a multifaceted intervention in an integrated deliver system. *J Gen Intern Med.* 2007;23:379–382.

21. Di Censo A, Guyatt G. Interpreting levels of evidence and grades of health care recommendations. In Di Censo A, Guyatt G, Ciliska D (eds), *Evidence Based Nursing. A Guide to Clinical Practice.* St. Louis, MO: Elsevier Mosby. 2005.

22. Haase A, Follmann M, Skipka G, Kirchner H. Developing search strategies for clinical practice guidelines in SUMSearch and Google Scholar and assessing their retrieval performance. *BMC Med Res Methodol.* 2007;7:28. http://www.pubmedcentral.nih.gov/articlerender.fcgi?artid=1925105

23. Wilczynski NL, Haynes RB, Lavis JN, et al. HSR Hedges team. Optimal search strategies for detecting health services research studies in MEDLINE. *CMAJ.* 2004;171:1179–1185. http://www.pubmedcentral.nih.gov/articlerender.fcgi?tool=pubmed&pubmedid=15534310

12

Secondary Publications: Economic Analyses

Angela Eady and Nancy Wilczynski

INTRODUCTION

Resources in health care are unavoidably finite and this has highlighted the importance of decisions about resource allocation. Health care professionals may participate in such decisions, which means they have to consider not only the effectiveness but also the costs of the screening (mammograms for breast cancer), diagnostic (magnetic resonance imaging for multiple sclerosis), therapeutic (defibrillators for coronary heart disease), and preventive (assertiveness training programs to prevent teen pregnancy) interventions they choose. One tool that helps delineate the benefits and costs of a health care procedure or treatment is an **economic analysis**, which uses formal quantitative methods to compare alternative interventions for their resource use and the outcomes achieved. Ideally, economic analyses can help to identify wasteful, ineffective procedures and less-costly interventions that are as effective as the high-cost ones.[1] The task is often more complex than it seems, however, because more effective interventions may be more costly, and certain tradeoffs have to be considered. Not surprisingly then, the number of economic analyses in the health care literature has grown over the years.[2]

Various types of economic analyses are used; high-quality ones have some common elements:

- First, they compare alternative strategies of screening, treatment, prevention, quality improvement, or diagnosis; doing nothing may be considered an alternative strategy.
- Second, they include data on costs and benefits, both of which are required for a full economic comparison. If only costs are included, the comparison is called a **cost analysis**, and it does not help in

formulating decisions about whether the intervention is an effective use of resources.

- Third, good economic analyses inform readers of the additional (or incremental) costs and benefits of 1 intervention over another.

Although good economic analyses share certain elements, they may differ in many other ways; e.g., design, methods, type of costs used, and the perspective taken when comparing costs and benefits. Some economic analysts have used a cube drawing to represent 3 dimensions of a health economic analysis: the types of analysis, costs and benefits, and the point of view from which an economic analysis is done.[3] The cube drawing shows that all of these aspects intersect and must be considered in relation to each another. These dimensions are discussed below after the clinical example. The design, or overall structure, of economic analyses will also be discussed.

The differences across economic analyses arise from the decisions that investigators make when doing an analysis. When analyzing costs and benefits for an intervention in a particular population, investigators often make assumptions about costs or benefits, and these may vary across different situations. In good economic analyses, *sensitivity analyses* will be used to see whether these assumptions, or changes in the assumptions, have an influence on the results.

CLINICAL EXAMPLE

Simon and colleagues[4] conducted a study to evaluate the incremental cost and cost-effectiveness (defined below) of a systematic treatment program in outpatients with diabetes mellitus. They noted that depression co-occurring with diabetes was associated with higher health services costs, suggesting that more effective depression treatment might reduce the use of other medical services. To investigate this possibility they conducted a randomized controlled trial comparing a systematic depression treatment program with usual care; 329 adult outpatients with diabetes mellitus and a current depressive disorder participated. Specialized nurses delivered a 12-month, stepped-care depression treatment program beginning with either problem-solving treatment psychotherapy or a structured antidepressant pharmacotherapy program. Subsequent treatment (combining psychotherapy and medication, adjustments to medication, and specialty referral) was adjusted according to clinical response. The main outcome measures were depressive symptoms assessed by blinded telephone interviews at 3, 6, 12, and 24 months, and health service costs determined using health plan accounting records. Over the 24-month follow-up period, patients assigned to the intervention group (systematic depression treatment program) had a mean of 61 additional days free of depression. They also had outpatient health services costs (i.e., outpatient services provided or purchased by

Group Health Cooperative as well as all services provided by intervention staff) that averaged $314 less when compared with patients in the usual care group. When an additional day free of depression was valued at $10, the net economic benefit of the intervention was $952 per patient treated. The authors concluded that for adults with diabetes mellitus and a current depressive disorder, systematic depression treatment increased the time free of depression and had economic benefits from the health plan perspective.

METHODOLOGICAL ISSUES

Economic Analysis Designs

Designs for economic analyses include: randomized controlled trials (as in our clinical example above); systematic reviews of cost-effectiveness analyses; retrospective analyses of a published randomized controlled trial; and decision models that use data from trials or systematic reviews to estimate the outcomes for a hypothetical group of patients. When data from previously published trials are used in an economic analysis, the methodology of those studies will influence the validity of the economic analysis.

Types of Economic Analyses

How interventions are compared in an analysis will depend on the way benefits and costs are measured and valued.[5] As has already been mentioned, a cost analysis, which may also be called a *cost minimization analysis*[5] or a *cost identification analysis*[3] considers costs only. This type of analysis is fairly basic, and is only useful insofar as the intervention is known to be equivalent or superior to the comparison intervention. In these cases, a cost analysis can show whether an effective intervention is less costly than interventions used in standard care. For example, Covinsky and colleagues compared the costs of caring for medical patients on a special unit designed to help older people maintain or achieve independence in self-care activities with the costs of usual care.[6] They used a randomized controlled trial and reported the health outcomes as well. Patients in the special unit spent less time in the hospital and were less likely to need home nursing. The readmission rates and caregiver strain scores were similar for both groups of patients. Given that the special unit was more effective for improving some outcomes and similar to standard care for all other outcomes, the costs can be compared. The authors found that the 2 interventions did not differ substantially in costs ($6608 total cost to care for patients in the special unit, compared with $7240 total cost to care for patients on the usual-care ward).

More often, though, new therapies, diagnostic tests, or health care procedures are more effective *and* more expensive. For analyzing the costs and benefits of these interventions (and for including data on benefits as well as costs), a finer level of analysis is required. Cost-benefit analyses, cost-effectiveness analyses, and cost-utility analyses are more sophisticated methods of comparing costs and benefits.

A **cost-benefit analysis** expresses all costs and benefits in monetary terms. The difference between the benefit (in monetary units) and the costs is called the *net benefit*. Interventions are considered favorable when their benefits exceed their costs (i.e., a positive net benefit). For example, Golaszewski and colleagues did a cost-benefit analysis of a major health program in the workplace called the "Taking Care Program."[7] The Travelers Insurance Company introduced this program to its 36,000 employees and retirees in the United States. The program consisted of a health risk appraisal, medical reference text, monthly health newsletter, several program introduction videotapes, and media blitzes (called "FOCUS programs") on selected health topics. Employees helped to implement the program. Golaszewski and colleagues calculated the costs of the program and translated the benefits into costs. They did this by estimating the costs of health care, absenteeism, death benefits that were paid out by the company, productivity gains, and income generated by the program through membership fees. They found that the Taking Care Program led to a net value—the total program effects minus costs—of $72.35 million, which translated into a benefit-cost ratio of 3:4.

Researchers often find it difficult to express outcomes in health care as monetary values. Cost-effectiveness and cost-utility analyses allow researchers to analyze benefits and costs without having to convert benefits into monetary values, and consequently these are more common in the health care literature.[2] The choice of a cost-effectiveness or cost-utility analysis will depend on the types of outcomes of interest.

If the interventions have the same health outcome, then a **cost-effectiveness analysis** can be done. It shows what the additional cost is for the additional improvement in health achieved by using 1 intervention rather than another. For example, Salzmann and colleagues wanted to determine whether it would be cost effective to extend screening recommendations to include mammograms for women 40 to 49 years of age.[8] The outcome in this study was reduced mortality, which was measured for 3 screening strategies. The authors did a cost-effectiveness analysis to compare the cost per life saved for biennially screening women from 50 to 69 years of age compared with: (1) no screening and (2) screening women every 18 months from 40 to 49 years of age, followed by screening biennially from 50 to 69 years age. They found that screening women 50 years and older cost $21,400 for each year of life saved, whereas extending screening to include women 40 to 49 years of age cost $105,000 for each year of life saved.

Interventions can affect patients' quality of life as well as their health outcomes. The different effects of an intervention make it difficult to do a cost-effectiveness analysis. In these instances, **cost-utility analyses** are used, which incorporate patient preferences for the types of interventions that are being compared. Cost-utility analyses report the number of years of life saved, which are adjusted for quality (these are also known as quality adjusted life years [QALY] gained). Glennie interviewed 7 patients with schizophrenia to collect data on patient preferences for the use of clozapine and risperidone compared with haloperidol.[9] She found that risperidone led to $6500 saved per year with a gain of 0.04 QALY, and clozapine led to $39,000 saved per year with a gain of 0.04 QALY. Cost-utility can be thought of as the nonmonetary "value" that an individual or society places on something.

Although economic analysts distinguish among the 4 different types of analysis, the terminology for economic analyses in the health care literature is not so neatly classified. The label of cost-benefit analysis is applied broadly. In a review of studies in MEDLINE, *Current Contents*, and HealthSTAR, Zarnke and colleagues found that 53% of the 95 studies that were labeled as cost-benefit analyses did not evaluate health outcomes.[10] Also, only 32% of the 95 studies were bona fide cost-benefit analyses; ie, health outcomes were translated into monetary values in them.

TYPES OF COSTS

Various costs are associated with the use of an intervention––some obvious and some less so. The types of costs included in an economic analysis will depend on the perspective taken, which is discussed in the next section. Costs can be classified as direct or indirect. **Direct costs** include costs of providing medical care (e.g., intervention costs and the health care professionals' salaries) and nonmedical costs to patients and families (e.g., patients' cost of transportation to the medical facility, and other such costs associated with illness and the receipt of medical care). **Indirect costs** include the broader costs of illness (e.g., time lost from work) or mortality (e.g., premature death leading to removal of that person from the workforce).

Economic analyses describe the types of costs and how they are measured. Changes in the value of money over time are taken into consideration. For some interventions, like screening, the benefits occur in the future. To determine the present value of these future costs, discount rates are used. Generally, these discount rates range from 2% to 6%. Salzmann and colleagues report that they included 3 costs in their analysis of breast cancer screening strategies: the cost of screening mammographic examinations, the cost of evaluating abnormal mammograms, and the cost of treating breast cancer.[8] These direct costs were measured in U.S. dollars, which were inflated to 1995 dollars by using the consumer price index for medical services. The authors also discounted costs at a rate of 3% per year. Rosenheck and colleagues included nonmedical costs in their study on clozapine in patients with schizophrenia, which were the costs of the criminal justice system (police contacts and arrests) and the administrative costs of transfer payments (programs that provide welfare or disability payments to patients).[11] Indirect costs were also included: loss of productivity (loss of earnings from employment) and family burden (days lost by family members from work and from unpaid domestic activity because of caring for the patient). They found that clozapine was more effective than haloperidol for patients with schizophrenia, with similar costs for both drugs. However, as Jones pointed out in a commentary, costs to the community may grow as patients with schizophrenia get better and start using services that were not of benefit to them before.[12] An economic analysis that includes the costs of community services would need to be done to see whether societal costs are increased by the use of clozapine.

THE PERSPECTIVE OF AN ECONOMIC ANALYSIS

Economic analyses are always done from a particular viewpoint. The perspective can be that of the patient, the payer, the health care provider, or society. The cost effectiveness of an intervention can change when analyzed from a different perspective. For example, when Anis and colleagues analyzed the cost effectiveness of cyclosporine in patients with rheumatoid arthritis from the perspective of the Ontario Ministry of Health (payer), they found that the incremental cost of using cyclosporine rather than placebo was $11,547 per patient each year.[13] From a societal perspective, however, the incremental cost was greater: $20,698 per patient each year. Some of the costs included in the analysis from the societal perspective were over-the-counter medication costs, the cost of home- visiting nurse services, and time lost from work.

TESTING THE ASSUMPTIONS OF AN ECONOMIC ANALYSIS

Economic analysts often make assumptions. These assumptions may include costs, the methods used to measure an outcome, discount rates, and estimates of the intervention's effect. The assumptions inherent in an economic analysis may influence the results, and show that it is sensitive to certain factors. A **sensitivity analysis** will help determine whether the results of an economic analysis are consistent or whether they require certain assumptions to be true. An economic model is often constructed, which allows sensitivity analyses to be repeated to determine the effect of varying assumptions or costs (e.g., differences in salaries or costs of drugs). Sometimes economic analysts will use the 95% confidence intervals (CIs) associated with the effects of an intervention to determine whether the results remain the same across different estimates of the effect.

In an economic analysis by Lave and colleagues, 3 different depression treatments were compared: psychotherapy, drug treatment (nortriptyline), and usual care by a primary care physician.[14] The authors calculated the cost for each additional depression-free day experienced by patients using the results from 1 of 2 scales to measure depression. They found that psychotherapy and nortriptyline were both more effective and more expensive than usual care. However, when they used the results from the second depression scale in the analysis, the effect was no longer statistically significant for psychotherapy. The analysis was sensitive to the type of scale used to measure depression.

SUMMARY

Economic analyses analyze the costs in relation to the benefits of an intervention. Data on benefits *and* costs are important for evaluating whether an intervention is an effective and efficient use of resources. Economic analyses should compare alternative strategies for diagnosis, therapy, prevention, or quality improvement, and they should also provide information about the additional, or incremental, costs and benefits of using one strategy (or intervention) over another. The methods used to evaluate the benefits of an intervention will influence its validity, which means that the trials or reviews used to obtain data should meet the criteria for therapy, diagnosis, or quality improvement trials, depending on which intervention is being studied. Different types of costs—direct and indirect—are used in economic analyses. The different methods of analyzing costs in relation to benefits are cost analyses (costs only are considered, so this type of analysis is useful only when the effectiveness of an intervention is known to be equivalent or superior to the alternative); cost-benefit analyses (the costs and benefits of an intervention are measured by using monetary values); cost-effectiveness analyses (the cost of the additional health improvement is calculated); and cost-utility analyses (the patient's quality of life is incorporated into the analysis, and the cost for each QALY is calculated). The health care literature does not differentiate clearly among cost analyses, cost-benefit analyses, and cost-effectiveness analyses. Economic analysts make assumptions about many aspects of an analysis, including costs and benefits; and when uncertainty exists in an economic analysis, sensitivity analyses are used to determine whether the results depend on certain assumptions being true. Economics also plays a major role in the production of health technology assessment reports that policy and decision makers use in making recommendations for implementation of services (see Chapter 13).

SEARCHING METHODOLOGY

Now that we have summarized the components of economic studies we move on to searching for economic studies in the large electronic databases such as MEDLINE. This task can be challenging but using search terms that target the methodology specific to economic studies in addition to your content terms (eg, diabetes and depression) can aid in retrieval effectiveness. The search terms available to use in 4 large electronic databases follow. The terms were compiled during the Clinical Hedges Study[15] after seeking input from clinicians and librarians in the United States and Canada. Index terms, subheadings, and publication types are assigned to each article in the database by staff working for the electronic database (eg, MEDLINE). Textwords are used to search for articles using the article title and the article abstract. Preferred search terms are shown for MEDLINE and EMBASE as search strategies were developed for detecting economic studies during the Clinical Hedges Study for these 2 databases.

MEDLINE

MeSH, Subheadings, Publication Types, and Textwords

MeSH (Medical Subject Headings — Index Terms)

Cost-benefit analysis*

Capital expenditures
"Costs and cost analysis"
Cost allocation
Cost control (can be exploded)
Cost savings
Cost of illness
Cost sharing (can be exploded)
Decision support techniques (can be exploded)
Decision trees
"Deductibles and coinsurance"
Direct service costs
Drug costs
Economics, hospital (can be exploded)
Economics, medical (can be exploded)
Economics, pharmaceutical
Economic value of life
Employer health costs
"Fees and charges" (can be exploded)

---

*Indicates a preferred term as determined in the Clinical Hedges Study.[16]

Fee-for-service plans
Fees, medical
Fees, pharmaceutical (can be exploded)
Health care costs (can be exploded)
Health care rationing
Health expenditures (can be exploded)
Health priorities
Health resources
Health services administration (can be exploded)
Health services research (can be exploded)
Hospital charges
Hospital costs
Life tables
Medical savings accounts
Models, economic (can be exploded)
Models, econometric
Markov chains
Monte Carlo method
Prepaid health plans
Prescription fees
Quality-adjusted life years
"Rate setting and review"
Utilization review (can be exploded)

Subheadings

Economics

Publication Types

None

Textwords (Same List Is Used for All 4 Databases)

Cost*
Cost:*
Costs*
Cost effective*
Cost effective:*
Cost effectiveness*
Economic*
Randomized*
Sensitivity analys:*

Cost analys:

---

*Indicates a preferred term as determined in the Clinical Hedges Study.[16,17]

Cost benefit:
Cost benefit analys:
Cost containment
Cost control:
Cost effectiveness ratio
Cost estimate:
Cost identification analys:
Cost minimization analys:
Cost minimisation analys:
Cost per life year sav:
Cost per life year estimate
Cost per life year gain:
Cost per patient:
Cost per QALY
Cost per QALYs
Cost per QALY gain:
Cost per quality adjusted life year:
Cost per unit of benefit
Cost per year of life gain:
Cost per year life sav:
Cost sav:
Cost sharing
Direct cost:
Direct benefit:
Discount cost:
Discount benefit:
Discounted benefit:
Discounted cost:
Drug cost:
Decision analys:
Decision analytic model:
Decision model:
Economic:
Economic evaluation:
Economic analys:
Economic assessment:
Economic model:
Expens:
Expensive
Expenditure:
Health care cost:
Health care expenditure:
Health resource allocation
Health resource utilization

Health resource utilisation
Health services research
Health service research
Hospital cost:
Indirect benefit:
Indirect cost:
Incremental:
Incremental analys:
Incremental cost:
Incremental cost effectiveness
Incremental cost effectiveness ratio
Incremental cost per life year
Incremental cost per life year gain:
Incremental cost per life year:
Incremental cost per QALY:
Incremental cost per QALY gain:
Life table
Life table method
Life year gain:
Life years gain:
Life year sav:
Life years sav:
Markov
Markov model:
Monte Carlo simulations method
Monte Carlo simulation method:
Monte Carlo simulation:
Modeling
Modelling
Net benefit:
Opportunity cost:
Pharmacoeconomic:
Per life year sav:
Per life year estimate
Per life year gain:
Per year of life sav:
Per unit of benefit
QALY
QALYs
Quality adjusted life year:
Quality adjusted life years gain:
Resource consumption
Sav:
Sensitivity analys:

Simulation
Simulator
Utilization review:
Utilisation review:
Years of life gain:
Years of life sav:

CINAHL (CUMULATIVE INDEX TO NURSING AND ALLIED HEALTH LITERATURE)

Index Terms, Subheadings, and Publication Types

Index Terms

Capitation fee
Comparative studies
Cost benefit analysis
Cost control (can be exploded)
Cost of living
Cost savings
"Costs and cost analysis" (can be exploded)
Data anlysis, statistical
Decision making
Economic aspects of illness
Economic value of life
Economics, pharmaceutical
Economics (can be exploded)
Fee for service plans
"Fees and charges" (can be exploded)
Funding source
Health care costs (can be exploded)
Health resource allocation
Health resource utilization
Health services administration (can be exploded)
"Health services needs and demand"
Health services research (can be exploded)
Hospital changes
Hospital costs
Insurance, health, reimbursement
Life table method
Long term care
Managed care programs
Medicare

Models, statistical
Nursing costs
Patient care (can be exploded)
Quality of life (can be exploded)
"Rate setting and review"
Reimbursement mechanisms
Resource allocation (can be exploded)
Utilization review (can be exploded)

Subheadings

None

Publication Types

None

EMBASE

Index Terms, Subheadings, and Publication Types

Index Terms

Cost effectiveness analysis*

Capitation fee
Cost benefit analysis
Cost control
Cost effectiveness analysis
Cost minimization analysis
Cost of illness
Cost (can be exploded)
Data analysis
Decision making
Decision theory
Disease simulation
Drug cost
Economic aspect (can be exploded)
Economic evaluation (can be exploded)
Economics (can be exploded)

---

*Indicates a preferred term as determined in the Clinical Hedges Study.[17]

Fee (can be exploded)
Health care cost (can be exploded)
Health care delivery (can be exploded)
Health care facilities and services (can be exploded)
Health care organization (can be exploded)
Health care planning
Health care policy
Health care system (can be exploded)
Health economics (can be exploded)
Health insurance (can be exploded)
Health service (can be exploded)
Health services research
Hospital billing
Hospital charge
Hospital cost (can be exploded)
Hospital finance
Hospital purchasing
Life expectancy
Life table
Medical fee
Model (can be exploded)
Nonbiological model
Occupational accident
Pharmacoeconomics (can be exploded)
Probability
Quality adjusted life year
Quality of life (can be exploded)
Simulation (can be exploded)
Simulator
Socioeconomics (can be exploded)
Statistical model
System analysis
Utilization review

Subheadings

None

Publication Types

None

PsycINFO

Index Terms, Subheadings, and Publication Types

Index Terms

"Costs and cost analysis" (can be exploded)
Cost containment
Decision support systems
Economics
Estimation (can be exploded)
Fee for service
Funding
Health care administration (can be exploded)
Health care costs
Health care services (can be exploded)
Health care utilization
Life expectancy
Markov chains
Mathematical modeling (can be exploded)
Professional fees (can be exploded)
Resource allocation
Response cost
Simulation (can be exploded)

Subheadings

None

Publication Types

None

EXAMPLES OF TEXTWORDS AND INDEXING USING OUR CLINICAL EXAMPLE

Citation for Our Clinical Example

Simon GE, Katon WJ, Lin EH, et al. Cost-effectiveness of systematic depression treatment among people with diabetes mellitus. *Arch Gen Psychiatry*. 2007;64:65–72.

Textwords and Index Terms Used in Our Clinical Example

Textwords (in the Title and Abstract of the Article)

Cost*
Costs*
Economic*
Cost-effectiveness

MEDLINE INDEXING

Cost-benefit analysis*
Health care costs
Economics (Subheading)
Prepaid health plans

EMBASE INDEXING

Cost effectiveness analysis*
Cost minimization analysis
Cost of illness
Health care cost
Health service

PROVEN STRATEGIES

Search Strategies (Filters) Derived during the Clinical Hedges Study [16,17]

Filter	MEDLINE (Ovid syntax)	EMBASE (Ovid syntax)
Sensitive	costs.tw. OR cost effective.tw. OR economic.tw.	cost effectiveness analysis.sh. OR randomized.tw. OR economic.tw.
Specific	cost effective.tw. OR sensitivity analys:.tw.	cost effectiveness.tw. OR sensitivity analys:.tw.
Minimize difference between Sensitivity and Specificity	cost-benefit analysis.sh. OR costs.tw. OR cost effective.tw.	cost.tw. OR costs.tw.

*See the Introduction for a description of how to use these filters and where to find them in Ovid and PubMed.

*Indicates a preferred term as determined in the Clinical Hedges Study.[16,17]

LINKS TO OTHER RESOURCES

Link to information regarding the Clinical Hedges Study http://hiru.mcmaster.ca/hiru/HIRU_Hedges_home.aspx

Link to how to use an article about economics:http://www.cche.net/users-guides/economic.asp

EXERCISES

Note that the search possibilities (answers) are detailed in the Appendix.

1. Is aspirin cost effective in the primary prevention of cardiovascular disease in women?
2. Is an adjuvant treatment course of spa treatment compared with usual care only cost effective in patients with fibromyalgia syndrome?

REFERENCES

1. Drummond M. Evidence-based medicine and cost-effectiveness: uneasy bedfellows [EBM Note]. *Evidence-Based Medicine.* 1998;3:133.
2. Elixhauser A, Halpern M, Schmier J, Luce BR. Health care CBA and CEA from 1991 to 1996: an updated bibliography. *Med Care.* 1998;36(5 Suppl):MS1–9.
3. Schulman KA, Glick HA, Yabroff KR, Eisenberg JM. Introduction to clinical economics: assessment of cancer therapies. *J Natl Cancer Inst Monogr.* 1995;19:1–19.
4. Simon GE, Katon WJ, Lin EH, et al. Cost-effectiveness of systematic depression treatment among people with diabetes mellitus. *Arch Gen Psychiatry.* 2007;64:65–72.
5. O'Brien B. Principles of economic evaluation for health care programs. *J Rheumatol.* 1995;22:1399–1402.
6. Covinsky KE, King JT Jr, Quinn LM, et al. Do acute care for elders units increase hospital costs? A cost analysis using the hospital perspective. *J Am Geriatr Soc.* 1997;45:729–734.
7. Golaszewski T, Snow D, Lynch W, et al. A benefit-to-cost analysis of a work-site health promotion program. *J Occup Med.* 1992;34:1164–1172.
8. Salzmann P, Kerlikowske K, Phillips K. Cost-effectiveness of extending screening mammography guidelines to include women 40 to 49 years of age. *Ann Intern Med.* 1997;127:955–965.
9. Glennie J. Technology overview: pharmaceuticals: pharmacoeconomic evaluations of clozapine in treatment-resistant schizophrenia and risperidone in chronic schizophrenia. Ottawa: Canadian Coordinating Office for Health Technology Assessment (CCOHTA): 1997 Jul.
10. Zarnke KB, Levine MA, O'Brien BJ. Cost-benefit analyses in the health care literature: don't judge a study by its label. *J Clin Epidemiol.* 1997;50:813–822.
11. Rosenheck R, Cramer J, Xu W, et al. A comparison of clozapine and haloperidol in hospitalized patients with refractory schizophrenia. Department of Veterans Affairs Cooperative Study Group on Clozapine in Refractory Schizophrenia. *N Engl J Med.* 1997;337:809–815.

12. Jones P. Commentary on "Clozapine reduced symptoms and side effects in patients who had refractory schizophrenia." *Evidence-Based Mental Health*. 1998;1:82. [Comment on: Rosenheck R, Cramer J, Xu W, et al. A comparison of clozapine and haloperidol in hospitalized patients with refractory schizophrenia. . Department of Veterans Affairs Cooperative Study Group on Clozapine in Refractory Schizophrenia. *N Engl J Med*. 1997;337:809–815.]

13. Anis AH, Tugwell PX, Wells GA, Stewart DG. A cost effectiveness analysis of cyclosporine in rheumatoid arthritis. *J Rheumatol*. 1996;23:609–616.

14. Lave JR, Frank RG, Schulberg HC, Kamlet MS. Cost-effectiveness of treatments for major depression in primary care practice. *Arch Gen Psychiatry*. 1998;55:645–651.

15. Wilczynski NL, Morgan D, Haynes RB; Hedges Team. An overview of the design and methods for retrieving high-quality studies for clinical care. *BMC Med Inform Decis Mak*. 2005;5:20.

16. Wilczynski NL, Haynes RB, Lavis JN, Ramkissoonsingh R, Arnold-Oakley AE; HSR Hedges team. Optimal search strategies for detecting health services research studies in MEDLINE. *CMAJ*. 2004;171:1179–1185.

17. McKinlay RJ, Wilczynski NL, Haynes RB; Hedges Team. Optimal search strategies for detecting cost and economic studies in EMBASE. *BMC Health Serv Res*. 2006;6:67.

13

Secondary Publications: Health Technology Assessment

Ann McKibbon

INTRODUCTION

Health technology assessment (HTA) documents are produced to provide a formal assessment for policy makers and administrators of the benefits and harms of an intervention. The documents are often in the form of technical reports rather than journal articles. They include a formal assessment of the harms and benefits associated with the "technology" along with a formal economic evaluation. The assessment of the technology's benefits and harms is a systematic review or meta-analysis of the literature. In many instances the HTA documents also include a model that can be used to project costs and benefits if that technology were to be implemented by a hospital, health maintenance organization, or other jurisdiction. Many countries with socialized medicine such as Canada and the United Kingdom, and much of Europe use HTA reports in their decision making to allow coverage for the people in their jurisdictions.

"Technology" is loosely defined. Most often things such as machinery and information technology (eg, magnetic resonance imaging, litotriptors) are studied. Other such interventions as various fertility treatments, cholesterol lowering agents, robotic surgery, and coronary stents impregnated with antibiotics are also studied and evaluated. The Canadian Agency for Drugs and Technology in Health defines technology as:

Health technology includes any method or intervention that is used to promote health; prevent, diagnose, or treat disease; or improve rehabilitation and long-term care. Technologies include drugs, devices, diagnostic agents, equipment, and medical and surgical procedures.

> **The definition also includes organizational and service systems that provide health care, such as telehealth.[1]**

Although HTA documents are designed for policy makers, they are also used by clinicians. The strength of an HTA is the foundational review of the literature. This systematic review of the literature is the basis for assessment of the risks and benefits. It also underpins the economic evaluation and modeling projections. HTA documents can provide the kind of reliable synthesized data that can go into the production of clinical practice guidelines (Chapter 12: Systematic Reviews).

CLINICAL EXAMPLE

Our clinical example for this chapter is respite care. Most health care provided outside the hospital setting is given to people over the age of 65 years, often by caregivers who look after spouses who have chronic and multiple conditions. The most common conditions are frailty, disability, cancer, and dementia.[2] In addition to spouses, care can be provided by other relatives, friends, and neighbors. The care given at home is often the patient's preference. Home care is substantially less costly to society than if the care were provided by nursing homes and other long-term facilities. One of the most important means of providing assistance to home care-givers is to provide occasional or routine respite care. Respite care is often given in the patient's home. The caregiver can then visit friends or relatives and recharge him- or herself. Respite care can also be provided by day care centers or by moving the patient to another home situation or an institution for a short period of time. Respite can be for an occasional weekend or week to provide an annual holiday for the caregiver. Respite care can also prepare the family and patient for eventual institutionalization. Common sense seems to say that respite care is good for the caregiver. It also probably keeps the patient at home longer and increases quality of life for everyone involved in the care situation.

Many people who are not self sufficient are cared for at home. This has tremendous cost and resource implications for individuals and society. The U.K. National Health Service (NHS) wanted to ascertain if respite care is cost effective; ie, do money and resources spent on providing respite care improve quality of life and reduce institutionalization to such an extent that the health care system should provide routine respite care for all who could benefit from it? The NHS also wanted to know what models of respite care exist in the United Kingdom and which are the most effective and cost effective. The NHS contracted with the Center for Health Economics at the University of York to produce an HTA report to address these issues.

The formal questions that the document was to address follow:

- **systematically to identify, appraise and synthesise the grey and published evidence for the effectiveness and cost-effectiveness of different models of community-based respite care for frail older people and their carers**
- **where data permits, to identify subgroups of carers and care recipients, for whom respite care is particularly effective or cost-effective**
- **to explore the practice, policy and research implications and to make recommendations for further research.**

The literature search comprised 37 databases and retrieval was limited to material published after 1980. Outcomes were related to the patient and caregivers and included quality of life, physical and mental health, satisfaction with care received, activities of daily living, caregiver burden, use of informal or volunteer services, use of any health and social services, time spent in care, and time to institutionalization. Respite care was defined to include day care, host family, in-home, institutional, and video respite. After bibliographies of review articles were checked for additional studies, 13,018 unique articles were included and 379 articles were screened using the full text of the articles. After review, 22 articles were included in the final analyses. Ten randomized controlled trials were included in these 22.

Results of the HTA report were somewhat disappointing for advocates of respite care. Much of the data came from the United States and other countries outside the United Kingdom. Satisfaction for caregivers receiving respite care was uniformly high across the studies. A small positive decrease in perceived caregiver burden and a small increase in their mental and physical health were seen. Little economic data were available from the studies and the identified studies provided little more that could be used for making economic conclusions or model building. The HTA report showed that more research is needed and suggested areas on which this research should concentrate.

HOW A HEALTH TECHNOLOGY ASSESSMENT REPORT IS DONE

Countries with socialized medicine rely heavily on information contained in HTA reports. Many of these countries have established regional and national organizations that are charged with producing these reports. For example, in Canada the first HTA organization was started in the province of Quebec in 1988.[3] By 2001, 1 national and 5 provincial agencies produced HTA reports,[4] totaling 187 reports during this time period. In 2000–2001, budgets ranged from $0.6 to $2.4 million in Canadian dollars. Ten to

35 people worked at each center. Assessment of 6 of the reports showed that acting on their recommendations the health care system saved approximately $15 million.[4] Overall the agencies saved the Canadian health care system between $16 million and $27 million per year. Many other countries feel that HTA agencies are equally effective. Because of health care financing differences in the United States, it has fewer HTA agencies with the U.S. Agency for Healthcare Research and Quality being a notable exception.

The Danish Centre for Health Technology Assessment publishes a handbook for the production of HTA reports.[6] It is available online and includes much information for HTA report producers and educators. The steps described in this document are similar to many of the process steps of methods for gathering and analyzing published information we have seen in many of our other chapters.

1. **Clarification of the policy issue in question**. As in our discussion of respite care, substantial health care resources were being consumed by those who accessed various forms of respite care. Little formal evidence was available to ascertain if respite care was effective and cost effective, or which form was best for individuals and the health care system. This situation of lack of evidence for common practices is common in our health care sytem.
2. **Formulation of the HTA question** that is acceptable to all parties involved including decision and policy makers and the health care institutions and professionals involved.
3. **Collection and analysis of the evidence** taking into account the technology and its various forms, the organizations involved, patients needs and preferences, and the economy and economic considerations.
4. **Synthesis of the evidence** and tailoring it to the situation and patients.
5. **HTA report production and distribution**.

Policy makers appreciate evidence in a summarized format. Consequently, many HTA reports include both abstracts and executive summaries, as well as the full evidence summaries and economic models. Many HTA reports are full technical reports that consist of several hundred or even thousands pages. Most HTA reports are not indexed in the major databases and therefore not easily found using traditional search methods.

METHODOLOGICAL ISSUES

Methodological issues for HTA report production and use relate to many other chapters. Many HTA reports use evidence from randomized controlled trials (Chapter 2: Therapy). All high-quality HTA documents include economics data (Chapter 12: Economics) and synthesis of existing evidence (Chapter 10: Systematic Reviews). Therefore we will not include methods on information retrieval for these aspects of HTA production in this chapter. In brief, an HTA is looking to answer the questions of does this technology work, for whom, at what cost (broadly based), and how does it compare with alternatives?

MEDLINE

MeSH, Subheadings, Publication Types, and Textwords

MeSH (Medical Subject Headings — Index Terms)

Benchmarking
Biomedical technology (can be exploded)
Biotechnology (can be exploded)
Cost and cost analysis (can be exploded)
Decision making (can be exploded)
Economics
Evaluation studies as topic
Evidence based practice
Health care delivery (can be exploded)
Health care policy and organization (can be exploded)
Health care rationing
Health care reform
Health policy (can be exploded)
Health services research
Medical informatics applications (can be exploded)
Models, economic
National health programs
Program evaluation (can be exploded)
Quality assurance, health care (can be exploded)
Quality control
Quality of health care
Resource allocation (can be exploded)
Technology (can be exploded)
Technology assessment, biomedical (can be exploded)
Technology transfer
Technology, dental
Technology, high-cost
Technology, medical
Technology, pharmaceutical
Technology, radiologic
Validation studies as topic

Subheadings

Standards and numerical data

Publication Types

None

CINAHL (CUMULATTIVE INDEX TO NURSING AND ALLIED HEALTH LITERATURE)

Index Terms, Subheadings, and Publication Types

Index Terms

Benchmarking
Biotechnology
Costs and cost analysis (can be exploded)
Cost benefit analysis
Decision making
Economics (can be exploded)
Evaluation (can be exploded)
Evaluation research (can be exploded)
Evidence based practice
Health care delivery (can be exploded)
Health care reform
Health informatics (can be exploded)
Health policy (can be exploded)
Health resource allocation
Health services research (can be exploded)
Health services for the aged
Medical informatics
Models, theoretical
National health programs
Program evaluation
Quality assurance (can be exploded)
Quality control (technology)
Quality improvement (can be exploded)
Resource allocation
Technology (can be exploded)
Technology transfer
Technology, dental
Technology, medical
Technology, pharmaceutical
Technology, radiologic
Validation studies

Subheadings

Standards and numerical data

Publication Types

None

EMBASE

Index Terms, Subheadings, and Publication Types

Index Terms

Biomedical technology assessment
Biomtechnology
Clinical evaluation
Cost (can be exploded)
Decision making
Economics (can be exploded)
Evaluation
Evaluation and follow up (can be exploded)
Evaluation research
Evidence based practice
Health care cost (can be exploded)
Health care organization
Health care planning
Health care quality (can be exploded)
Health economics (can be exploded)
Health service
Hospital cost (can be exploded)
Medical technology
Model (can be exploded)
Performance measurement system
Planning (can be exploded)
Policy
Quality control (can be exploded)
Resource allocation
Resource management (can be exploded)
Surgical technology
Technology (can be exploded)

Subheadings

None

Publication Types

None

PsycINFO

Index Terms, Subheadings, and Publication Types

Index Terms

Cost containment
Costs and cost analysis (can be exploded)
Decision making (can be exploded)
Decision theory
Economics (can be exploded)
Evidence based practice (can be exploded)
Health care costs (can be exploded)
Health care delivery (can be exploded)
Health care services (can be exploded)
Heuristic modeling
Mathematical modeling
Mental health program evaluation
Policy making (can be exploded)
Resource allocation
Stochastic modeling
Technology (can be exploded)
Technology innovation
Technology transfer
Treatment effectiveness evaluation
Uncertainty (can be exploded)

Subheadings

None

Publication Types

None

INDEXING TERMS POSSIBLE

Textwords

See also chapters for Economics (Chapter 12), Systematic Reviews
(Chapter 10), and Clinical Practice Guidelines (Chapter 13) for suggestions
of additional textwords and index terms.

Health technology assessment
Health technology monitoring

HTA
Impact research
Technology assessment
Technology monitoring

EXAMPLES OF TEXTWORDS AND INDEXING USING OUR CLINICAL EXAMPLE

Textwords and Index Terms Used in Our Clinical Example

Citation for Our Clinical Example 1

Mason A, Weatherly H, Spilsbury K, Arksey H, Golder S, Adamson J, Drummond M, Glendinning C. A systematic review of the effectiveness and cost-effectiveness of different models of community-based respite care for frail older people and their carers. *Health Tech Assess.* 2007 Apr;11(15):1–157, iii.

Textwords (in the Title and Abstract of the Article)

Systematic review
Effectiveness
Cost effectiveness
Models
Review the evidence

MEDLINE INDEXING

Statistics and numerical data (subheading)
Health services for the aged
Health policy

CINAHL INDEXING

Health policy
Health services for the aged
Cost benefit analysis

EMBASE INDEXING

Cost effectiveness analysis
Economic evaluation
Health care quality
Health program
Patient satisfaction
Quality of life

Citation for Our Clinical Example 2

Ospina MB, Bond K, Karkhaneh M, Tjosvold L, Vandermeer B, Liang Y, Bialy L, Hooton N, Buscemi N, Dryden DM, Klassen TP. Meditation practices for health: state of the research. *Evid Rep Technol Assess* (Full Rep). 2007 Jun;(155):1–263. No terms in the title or abstract.

MEDLINE INDEXING

Technology assessment, biomedical
Government agencies

Citation for Our Clinical Example 3

Perry S, Thamer M. Medical innovation and the critical role of health technology assessment. *JAMA*. 1999 Nov 17;282(19):1869–1872.

Textwords (in the Title and Abstract of the Article)

Health technology assessment (note no abstract)

MEDLINE INDEXING

Resource allocation
Technology assessment, biomedical

EMBASE INDEXING

Biomedical Technology Assessment
Clinical Practice
Cost Benefit Analysis
Decision Making
Health Care Cost
Health Care Policy

PROVEN STRATEGIES

No proven search filters for the large health databases are available for HTA reports. The most effective searching for HTA material is described in the following section.

LINKS TO OTHER RESOURCES

Many organizations provide access to HTA reports or information important to HTA producers. Much searching must be done in the gray literature as many reports are considered to be internal documents and dissemination efforts are often limited. Gray literature sites that describe methods and sites include the following.

- American Library Association. Association of College and Research Libraries. Gray literature: Resources for locating unpublished research. http://www.ala.org/ala/acrl/acrlpubs/crlnews/backissues2004/march04/graylit.cfm
- University of British Columbia. Libraries. Searching for Grey Literature. http://toby.library.ubc.ca/subjects/subjpage2.cfm?id=877

HTA specific web sites provide searching and related information. The first 2 sites that follow have a wealth of information related to HTA production and searching. The second 2 provide listings of completed and ongoing HTAs.

- Alberta Heritage Foundation for Medical Research. Health Technology Assessment on the Net: A Guide to Internet Sources of Information. Updated regularly. Dennett L, Chatterley T. [authors] 10th edition in 2008. http://www.ihe.ca/publications/library/2008/health-technology-assessment-on-the-net-10th/
- HTAi (Health Technology Assessment international) Vortal. This site is maintained by a large group of international librarians who are involved with HTA report production. http://216.194.91.140/vortal/
- CADTH Canadian Agency for Drugs and Technologies in Health. This site holds a wealth of information related to Canadian HTA production including a comprehensive list of completed and in progress HTAs. http://cadth.ca/index.php/en/hta
- York University. Centre for Reviews and Dissemination. Health Technology Assessment (HTA) Database. http://www.crd.york.ac.uk/crdweb/Home.aspx?DB=HTA&SessionID=&SearchID=&E=0&D=0&H=0&SearchFor= This site includes linkages to more than 7000 completed HTAs and related documents.

EXERCISE

Note that the search possibilities (answers) are detailed in the Appendix.

1. Determine how many counties have completed HTAs on the use of portable home dialysis units. Do they have conflicting recommendations?

REFERENCES

1. Canadian Agency for Drugs and Technology in Health. FAQ page. Accessed November 23, 2008. https://secure.cadth.ca/index.php/en/hta/faq

2. Mason A, Wetherly H, Spilsbury H, et al. A systematic review of the effectiveness and cost-effectiveness of different models of community-based respite care for frail older people and their carers. *Health Technol Assess.* 2007;11:1–157, iii.

3. Hailey DM. Health technology assessment in Canada: diversity and evolution. *Med J Aust.,* 2007;187:286–288.

4. Lehoux P, Tailliez S, Denis JL, Hivon M. Redefining health technology assessment in Canada: diversification of products and contextualization of findings. *Int J Technol Assess Health Care.* 2004;20:325–336.

5. McGregor M, Brophy JM. End-user involvement in health technology assessment (HTA) development: a way to increase impact. *Int J Technol Assess Health Care.* 2005; 21: 263–267.

6. Kristensen FB, Signund H. (editors). Health Technology Assessment Handbook. National Board of Health. Denmark. 2nd edition. 2008. Accessed August 23, 2008. http://www.dacehta.dk.

Glossary

The Glossary includes definitions for the terms used in the textbook. We have tried to use common-sense, easily understood definitions. Other sources will likely give alternate definitions so keep looking if our definition is not clear.

Term	Chapter	Definition
Absolute difference	2	This is the arithmetic difference between 2 numbers. This is often seen in comparing proportions of events in clinical trials.
Bias	2	An unintended influence on an outcome or process. Many biases exist. Biases can keep researchers from determining the truth in situations under study.
Blinding	2	Blinding happens when people involved with a study do not know group assignments (for therapy studies) or exposure or outcome status (for etiology studies). Those who can be blinded include the study participants, the health care professionals involved in the care of the participants, study personnel including the outcome assessors, data analysts, report writers, and sponsors.
Benefit	4	A measure of the "good" things that can happen because of a treatment or situation. *See also* Harm.
Case-control study	4	A study that starts with people who have the outcome of interest. Groups are formed, some of who have the outcome and some who do not have the outcome. They are often "marched" in pairs. Analysis looks back in time to ascertain if the people with the outcome have a higher rate of having the exposure than the people without the outcome.

(Continued)

Term	Chapter	Definition
Causation	4	*See* Etiology
Clinical decision rule	6	*See* Clinical prediction guide
Clinical practice guideline	11	Systematically derived set of actions and recommendations often based on evidence for certain clinical situations. They are often used to set standards of care to insure that patients get the care they need and not care they do not need.
Clinical prediction guide	6	A systematically developed statement designed to reduce the uncertainty in clinical decision making by defining how to use clinical findings to make predictions.
Clinical prediction rule	6	*See* Clinical prediction guide
Code breaking	2	Actions whereby people use various means to discover trial aspects to which they were not to know—i.e., foiling attempts at blinding.
Confidence interval	2	Confidence intervals (often abbreviated as CIs) are a statistical representation of the range of values that the outcome of a study could have taking into account the variation in the data. 95% CIs represent the range in values that one would expect if they were to repeat the trial 100 times using similar participants. 99% CIs and 90% CIs are also seen in the literature.
Cohort study	4	Cohort studies deal with "groups". Groups are defined at baseline and then followed forward in time to ascertain the outcomes. Can also use data collected previously. Strong methodology although not as strong as randomized controlled trials.
Collaborative review	10	A systematic review that combines not study-level data but data from each individual patient in each study.
Control group	2	The control group in various studies is the group that receives "standard" treatment or care. This can be active treatment such as drugs or placebo. The results of the control group are compared with the experimental or study group to draw conclusions.
Controlled clinical trial	2	*See* Randomized controlled trial

Cost analysis	12	Only costs are included. It does not help in formulating decisions about whether the intervention is an effective use of resources.
Cost identification analysis	12	*See* Cost analysis
Cost minimization analysis	12	*See* Cost analysis
Cost-benefit analysis	12	Expresses all costs and benefits in monetary terms. The difference between the benefit (in monetary units) and the costs is called the *net benefit*. Interventions are considered favorable when their benefits exceed their costs.
Cost-effectiveness analysis	12	If the interventions have the same health outcome, then a cost-effectiveness analysis can be done. It shows what the additional cost is for the additional improvement in health achieved by using one intervention rather than another.
Cost-utility analyses	12	Incorporates patient preferences for the types of interventions that are being compared. Cost-utility analyses report the number of years of life saved, which are adjusted for quality (these are also known as quality adjusted life years [QALY] gained).
Confounding factor	4	A confounding factor "acts" by affecting both the exposure and outcome. Presence of a confounder makes analysis and understanding of etiology questions complex and challenging. For example, smoking is often a confounder in drinking studies.
Criterion standard	3	*See* Gold standard.
Decision analysis	7	Practice that incorporates philosophy, technology, information science, methodology, and professional practice into decision making using formal methods. They incorporate multiple aspects of the decision, often using modeling to provide a decision and decision route for a given problem.
Decision tree	7	A graphical representation of all possible outcomes and the flow of the various sequential decisions and their outcomes, often factoring in the values of the person making the decision.
Diagnosis	3	The process of identifying a disease or condition in symptomatic patients by its signs and symptoms, or from the results of various diagnostic procedures (e.g., biopsy).

(Continued)

Term	Chapter	Definition
Diagnostic standard	3	*See* Gold standard.
Differential diagnosis	8	Involves the process of weighing the probability that one disease rather than another disease accounts for a patient's illness.
Direct costs	12	Includes costs of providing medical care (for example, intervention costs and the health care professionals' salaries) and nonmedical costs to patients and families (for example, patients' cost of transportation to the medical facility, and other such costs associated with illness and the receipt of medical care).
Disease manifestation	8	Findings the clinicians can gather directly from the patient, usually during the medical interview or physical examination.
Dummy	2	*See* Placebo
Economic analysis	12	Helps delineate the benefits and costs of a health care procedure or treatment and uses formal quantitative methods to compare alternative interventions for their resource use and outcomes achieved.
Ethnography	9	A type of qualitative study that seeks to learn about how people interpret their experience and adapt their behavior within the context of their own culturally defined environment.
Etiology	4	Etiology deals with the causes of a disease, condition, or situation.
False negative rate	3	The proportion of patients who received a negative test result when they do have the target disorder or disease.
False positive rate	3	The proportion of patients who received a positive test result when they do not have the target disorder or disease.
Forest plots	10	A pictorial plot of the studies that have gone into analyzing the articles in a systematic review/ meta-analysis. One row per study with a final row showing the final result from the analysis of the studies above.
Generalizable	2	A study is generalizable if the results of the study are strong enough and done carefully so that the findings can be applied with confidence to similar people who were not part of the original study.

Gold standard	3	Refers to the commonly accepted "proof" that the patient does or does not have the target disorder or disease of interest. The "gold" standard might be an autopsy or biopsy. The "gold" standard provides objective criteria (e.g., laboratory test not requiring interpretation) OR a current clinical standard (e.g., a venogram for deep venous thrombosis) for diagnosis.
Grounded theory	9	A type of qualitative study that set out to develop theory grounded in the real world of the participants.
Health Technology Assessment	13	Health Technology Assessment is a formal evaluation for policy and decision makers that assesses the benefits and harms of a health technology or intervention along with economic analyses. These are often summaries of the literature and done after standard clinical trials have shown benefits. More often used by policy makers than individual clinicians.
Harm	4	Deals with the side affects or problems associated with a treatment or other situation. Opposite of benefit.
Heterogeneity	10	The aspects of the items under consideration are different or dissimilar and should not be combined because of this dissimilarity.
Homogeneity	10	Consisting of similar parts or aspects. Articles that are homogeneous can be considered to be "combinable"
Inception cohort	5	"Inception" means early, uniformed point in time for the disease; and "cohort" means following a group of people forward in time.
Indirect costs	12	Includes the broader costs of illness (for example, time lost from work) or mortality (for example, premature death leading to removal of that person from the workforce).
Individual patient data meta-analysis	10	A meta-analysis (which see) that combines data at the individual patient level rather than data at the study level.
Influence diagram	7	A pictorial representation of a decision model. Useful for decisions that are too complex for a decision tree.
Intervention	2	Refers to a procedure or action that will potentially improve care. Nurses use the term interventions while physicians often use the terms therapy or treatment. These terms are equivalent.

(Continued)

Term	Chapter	Definition
Masking	2	*See* Blinding
Meta-analysis	10	Broad term that includes reports that collect and synthesize data from individual studies to provide new information—beyond summaries. Most often evaluate quantitative studies but can include qualitative studies also.
Meta-ethnography	9	*See* Meta-synthesis
Meta-synthesis	9	Results of multiple qualitative studies on a specific topic combined and analyzed in a systematic review
Narrative review	10	A review article that is not systematic. These reviews are often cover broad areas and written by an expert in the field. They are like textbook chapters. Students value these narrative reviews. *See also* Systematic reviews.
Natural history	5	The progression of untreated disease.
Negative likelihood ratio (-LR)	3	Incorporates both the sensitivity and specificity of the test and indicate how much the probability of disease changes from baseline when the test result is negative.
Negative predictive value	3	The proportion of patients with negative test results who do not have the disease or condition in question.
NNH	2	*See* Number needed to harm
NNT	2	*See* Number needed to treat
Number needed to harm	2	A calculation used to show how often adverse events happen in association with a treatment compared with an alternative. It shows how many people would have a certain adverse event during treatment to have one additional person show harms. The smaller the number the more often harm happens during the treatment.
Number needed to treat	2	A calculation used to show how effective a treatment is compared with an alternative. It shows how many people would have to be treated to have one additional person obtain benefit. The smaller the number the more effective is the treatment.
Odds ratio	4	The odds ratio is a measure of the likelihood that one was exposed to the risk factor (eg, spouse with higher education) now that one has the outcome (eg, one's own later or earlier death).

Patient decision aids	7	Tools that provide assistance to a person making a health care decision. They often present options and their rates of cure or improvement as well as adverse effects. Many systems also help the patient assess the value of the decisions and their personal preferences in regard to these outcomes and risks. These decision aids may be online or in paper format. The aids are designed to complement interactions with health professionals, not to replace them.
Phenomenology	9	A type of qualitative study concerned with describing the human or "lived" experience using the subjective or first-person experience as a source of knowledge.
Placebo	2	An intervention that is not "real" although most people in a trial often cannot tell the difference. Placeboes are most often used in drug studies where one group gets the medication and the other group gets inert substances designed to look, feel, taste and smell the same as the active agent. Also called "dummy" in UK trials.
Pooled data	10	Data that have been combined in a meta-analysis or similar synthesis.
Positive likelihood ratio (+LR)	3	Incorporates both the sensitivity and specificity of the test and indicate how much the probability of disease changes from baseline when the test result is positive.
Positive predictive value	3	The proportion of patients with positive test results who have the disease or condition in question.
Post-test odds	3	The odds that the patient has the target disorder or disease after the test is conducted. Calculated by multiplying pretest likelihood of having the disease by the +LR or −LR depending on whether the test result for the patient is positive or negative.
Pretest likelihood	3	*See* Prevalence.
Pretest probability	3	*See* Prevalence.
Prevalence (in diagnosis)	3	The proportion of patients with the target disorder or the disease in question among all tested patients. Prevalence is also sometimes called pretest probability or pretest likelihood of the target disorder, disease, or condition.

(Continued)

Term	Chapter	Definition
Prevention	2	Prevention is usually studied using a randomized controlled trial methodology. Primary prevention refers to trying to stop or prevent something like depression or teen pregnancy from happening for the first time. Secondary prevention deals with trying to stop something from happening again (e.g., a myocardial infarction). Tertiary prevention is a term used less often. It refers to trying to moderate or alleviate the adverse effects of a disease or disorder that cannot be cured or prevented.
Primary prevention	2	*See* Prevention
Prognosis	5	The progression of treated disease.
Publication bias	10	Publication bias is defined as studies with negative results (that is, that do not show an expected difference) have been shown to be submitted less often for publication, be submitted longer after completion of the study, be rejected more often by journal editors, and be published in less well known or in less respected journals than studies with "positive" results.
Purposeful sample	9	Selecting a sample of study participants based on their ability to meet the informational needs of the study.
p-value	2	Deals with the probability of getting a certain result or one that is more extreme. It can be taken to mean that the smaller the p-value, the more likely that the results did not happen by chance alone but because of the treatment or intervention given. A p-value below or less than 0.05 is considered to be the "dividing line" between effective and not effective treatments.
Qualitative research	9	The type of research that is done when you want to know about how people *feel* or *experience* certain situations.
Quality improvement	2	Studies that seek to show improvements in the process of care that are often also associated with improvements in outcomes also. May be educational interventions or physical changes in processes or staffing.

Randomized controlled trial	2	A research methodology whereby study participants are allocated to study groups using random allocation methods. Each group receives one of the therapies or interventions to be studied, one of which is often existing standard therapy (control group). The control group may also receive a placebo or sham intervention. After a preset period of time the groups are compared to determine the effects (and comparative effects) of the therapies studied so that decisions can be made to ascertain the most effective
Rate	2	How often something happens—often a proportion of those having an event compared with the whole group being considered.
Receiver operating characteristic curves	3	A graphical plot of sensitivity versus (1 − specificity).
Receiver operator characteristic curves	3	*See* Receiver operating characteristic curves.
Relative difference	2	A measure of the difference in rates or risk between groups assessed or divided by the baseline rate in the untreated or unexposed group. Can be relative risk or relative benefit.
Risk	2	On individual's chance of having an event occur.
ROC	3	*See* Receiver operating characteristic curves.
Screening	3	The process of identifying a disease or condition in asymptomatic patients from the results of various diagnostic procedures (e.g., mammography).
Secondary prevention	2	*See* Prevention
Secondary Publication	10	A secondary publication is one in which the investigators collect and analyze data from existing publications to produce summaries of the information or new information. Secondary publications include systematic reviews and meta-analyses, clinical practice guidelines, health technology assessment reports, and often economics studies.
Sensitivity	3	Measures the proportion of patients with the disease or disorder as defined by the gold standard who have a positive test result.

(*Continued*)

Term	Chapter	Definition
Sensitivity analysis	12	Will help determine whether the results of an economic analysis are consistent or whether they require certain assumptions to be true.
Sham	2	*See* Placebo
Specificity	3	Measures the proportion of patients without the disorder or condition as defined by the gold standard who have a negative test result.
Sub group analyses	2	Studies are designed to answer one main question and often several secondary questions. In addition, data analysis often shows the need for other analyses, such as differences between men and women. The analyses done to answer new questions or questions about part of the study group are called subgroup analyses.
Systematic review article	10	A systematic review is a review article that includes a definite question to address, the search methods including terms and databases used to identify material for inclusion, and inclusion and exclusion criteria for this material. Meta-analyses are a subclass of systematic reviews.
Technology assessment	12	*See* Health Technology Assessment
Tertiary prevention	2	*See* Prevention
Therapy	2	An action or intervention that can potentially improve care or prevent diseases or conditions. Nurses prefer the term intervention.
Treatment	2	*See* Therapy

Appendix

SEARCHING EXERCISES FOR CHAPTER 2

Therapy, Prevention and Control, and Quality Improvement

1. What evidence exists that individualized computer or internet advice is beneficial to those who wish to lose weight?

   Go to Clinical Queries in PubMed (http://www.ncbi.nlm.nih.gov/entrez/query/static/clinical.shtml) and enter the terms
   "Weight Loss (Computers or Internet)" in the search window under the section titled Search by clinical Study Category and hit the radio buttons for therapy and narrow, specific search. Click GO. Searching on January 15, 2009, 96 citations were found with many that seem to address this problem—looks like online tools play a role, although not a substantial one in weight reduction and maintenance.

2. How strong is the evidence that the establishment of safe injection sites (distribution of needles and provision of a location for people with major substance abuse problems) as described in British Columbia and Australia work at decreasing the spread of diseases?

   This is an important topic and no clinical trials seem to exist. Other kinds of evidence, with less strength exist, however.
   Go to PubMed (http://www.ncbi.nlm.nih.gov/entrez/query/static/clinical.shtml), put in the terms: "safer injecting facilities" or "safe injection sites" or "safer injecting facility" or "safe injection site." This gave 27 citations on January 15, 2009 showing some experience in Canada and the Netherlands for providing the service.

SEARCHING EXERCISES FOR CHAPTER 3

Diagnosis and Screening

1. Can short questionnaires be used to detect anxiety disorders in primary care?

   Go to the Clinical Queries page in PubMed (http://www.ncbi.nlm.nih. gov/entrez/query/static/clinical.shtml) and enter the terms "anxiety primary care" in the search window under the section titled Search by Clinical Study Category and hit the radio buttons for Diagnosis and Narrow, specific search. Click GO. Conducting this search on March 26, 2008, 66 citations are retrieved. Citation #3, PMID 17909240 addresses your question.

2. Can plasma fatty acid analysis be used in the diagnosis of cystic fibrosis?

   Go to the Clinical Queries page in PubMed (http://www.ncbi.nlm.nih. gov/entrez/query/static/clinical.shtml) and enter the terms "cystic fibrosis fatty acid" in the search window under the section titled Search by Clinical Study Category and hit the radio buttons for Diagnosis and Narrow, specific search. Click GO. Conducting this search on March 26, 2008, 6 citations are retrieved. None are on target. Return to the Clinical Queries page and enter the same search terms but broaden the search by hitting the radio buttons for Diagnosis and Broad, sensitive search. Conducting this search on March 26, 2008, 88 citations are retrieved. Citation #5, PMID 17130178 addresses your question.

SEARCHING EXERCISES FOR CHAPTER 4

Etiology, Causation, and Harm

1. Alzheimer disease is becoming more common—maybe because the baby boomers are getting older. Find all the risk factors you can: both factors that are protective and those associated with an increased risk. Grade the evidence you find according to the following categories:

   - Grade A Randomized controlled trials
   - Grade B Cohort studies
   - Grade C Case-control studies
   - Grade D Case series (five to 20 patients and no control group)
   - Grade E Case reports (one or two persons) and opinion

   This is a tremendously complex and controversial topic—and one that is not sorted out yet. Searching in Ovid Medline the use of the terms

"*Alzheimer disease/etiology" and "*Alzheimer disease/prevention and control" provide much information for consideration. Genetics, diabetes, and zinc consumption seem to increase the risk for Alzheimer disease while issues such as statins, antihypertension medication, and nonsteroidal anti-inflammatory agents; exercise; mental stimulation; higher education; and moderate wine consumption may play a role in prevention.

2. Health literacy seems to be an important topic. Does evidence exist that good health literacy is associated with improved mortality?

   The following suggestions use Ovid Technologies databases for retrieval. Note that CINAHL is no longer available through Ovid. Some cohort data seem to indicate that low health literacy levels are indeed associated with increased mortality. The next big question is to ascertain if improving health literacy levels will counter this increased mortality—issues of association and causation at their "best."

MEDLINE

health literacy.mp. and (exp *mortality.sh. or mo.fs.) and (exp case control study.sh. or exp prospective study.sh or exp retrospective study.sh. or cohort analysis.mp)

CINAHL

health literacy.tw. and exp *Mortality.sh. and (exp case control studies.sh. or correlational studies.sh. or cross sectional studies.sh. or exp prospective studies.sh.)

EMBASE

health literacy.mp. and exp *mortality.sh. and (exp case control study.sh. or exp prospective study.sh. or exp retrospective study.sh. or cohort analysis.mp.

SEARCHING EXERCISES FOR CHAPTER 5

Prognosis

1. What is the long-term prognosis of Crohn disease?

   Go to the Clinical Queries page in PubMed (http://www.ncbi.nlm.nih.gov/entrez/query/static/clinical.shtml) and enter the terms "crohn's disease" in the search window under the section titled Search by Clinical Study Category and hit the radio buttons for Prognosis and Narrow, specific search. Click GO. Conducting this search on April 16, 2008,

1012 citations are retrieved. Citation #134, PMID 17229220 addresses your question.

2. Are there factors that predict survival in patients with advanced esophageal cancer?

Go to the Clinical Queries page in PubMed (http://www.ncbi.nlm.nih. gov/entrez/query/static/clinical.shtml) and enter the terms "esophageal cancer" in the search window under the section titled Search by Clinical Study Category and hit the radio buttons for Prognosis and Narrow, specific search. Click GO. Conducting this search on April 16, 2008, 2881 citations are retrieved. Citation #54, PMID 18081735 addresses your question.

   This may seem like too many citations to retrieve. However, if you were to conduct this search without using the Clinical Queries you would retrieve 4782 citations if you searched using "esophageal cancer prognosis" in the main PubMed window and if you were to search using only "esophageal cancer" you would retrieve 28,402 citations.

SEARCHING EXERCISES FOR CHAPTER 6

Clinical Predication Guides

1. Is there a tool for predicting the probability of sentinel lymph node metastasis in breast cancer?

Go to the Clinical Queries page in PubMed (http://www.ncbi.nlm. nih.gov/entrez/query/static/clinical.shtml) and enter the terms "sentinel lymph node metastasis breast cancer" in the search window under the section titled Search by Clinical Study Category and hit the radio buttons for Clinical Prediction Guides and Narrow, specific search. Click GO. Conducting this search on May 29, 2008, 67 citations are retrieved. Several citations address your question including citation #1, PMID 18445838, citation #3, PMID 18303684, and citation #10, PMID 17664461.

2. Is there a tool to predict functional decline in older adults who have been discharged from the emergency department?

Go to the Clinical Queries page in PubMed (http://www.ncbi.nlm.nih. gov/entrez/query/static/clinical.shtml) and enter the terms "functional decline older adults" in the search window under the section titled Search by Clinical Study Category and hit the radio buttons for Clinical Prediction Guides and Narrow, specific search. Click GO. Conducting this search on May 29, 2008, 12 citations are retrieved. None of which appear relevant to your question.

Return to the Clinical Queries page enter the same search terms but broaden the search by hitting the ratio buttons for Clinical Prediction Guides and Broad, sensitive search. Conducting this search on March 29, 2008, 435 citations are retrieved. Citation #33 PMID 17661968 addresses your question.

SEARCHING EXERCISES FOR CHAPTER 7

Decision Analyses

1. For geriatric patients what diseases and conditions have been studied using formal decision analyses?

   This is a difficult search to do because of the issue of searching for geriatrics articles. Some material is found using PubMed and the following list of terms

   "decision analysis" decision support techniques (geriatrics or aged)

   The phrase "decision analysis" decision support techniques in PubMed seems to retrieve many of the formal decision analyses.

2. What do formal decision analyses say about treating otitis media in children with respect to antibiotics, tubes, and no treatment?

   Again in PubMed, put in "decision analysis" decision support techniques otitis media. We have not put in children as otitis media is generally considered to be a children's disease. Five citations were found on January 15, 2009, four of which seem to fit the question.

   1. Meropol SB. Valuing reduced antibiotic use for pediatric acute otitis media.Pediatrics. 2008 Apr;121(4):669-73. PMID: 18381529

   2. Higgins TS, McCabe SJ, Bumpous JM, Martinez S. Medical decision analysis: indications for tympanostomy tubes in RAOM by age at first episode. Otolaryngol Head Neck Surg. 2008 Jan;138(1):50-6. PMID: 18164993

   3. Manarey CR, Westerberg BD, Marion SA. Clinical decision analysis in the treatment of acute otitis media in a child over 2 years of age.J Otolaryngol. 2002 Feb;31(1):23-30.PMID: 11883437

   4. Bergus GR, Lofgren MM. Tubes, antibiotic prophylaxis, or watchful waiting: a decision analysis for managing recurrent acute otitis media. J Fam Pract. 1998 Apr;46(4):304-10.PMID: 9564372

SEARCHING EXERCISES FOR CHAPTER 8

Differential Diagnosis and Disease Manifestation

1. What is the differential diagnosis for unexplained drop attacks in older persons?

    Go to the Clinical Queries page in PubMed (http://www.ncbi.nlm.nih. gov/entrez/query/static/clinical.shtml) and enter the terms "drop attack*" in the search window under the section titled Search by Clinical Study Category and hit the radio buttons for Diagnosis and Narrow, specific search. Click GO. Conducting this search on June 5 2008, 2 citations are retrieved, none of which are relevant.

    Return to the Clinical Queries page enter the same search terms but broaden the search by hitting the ratio buttons for Diagnosis and Broad, sensitive search. Conducting this search on June 5, 2008, 125 citations are retrieved. Citation #26 PMID 15667379 addresses your question.

2. What is the clinical manifestation of Lyme disease in children?

    Go to the Main page in PubMed (http://www.ncbi.nlm.nih.gov/sites/ entrez) and enter the terms "manifestation lyme disease" in the search window. Click GO. Conducting this search on June 5, 2008, 313 citations are retrieved. Citation #3, PMID 18431910 addresses your question.

SEARCHING EXERCISES FOR CHAPTER 9

Qualitative

1. What are the experiences of inpatients who have pressure ulcers?

    Go to the Special Queries page in PubMed (http://www.nlm.nih.gov/ bsd/special_queries.html) and click on Health Services Research (HSR) Queries. Enter the terms "pressure ulcers" in the search window and hit the radio buttons for Qualitative and Narrow, specific search. Click GO. Conducting this search on May 6, 2008, 44 citations are retrieved. Citation #7, PMID 17419791 addresses your question.

2. What are the perceptions of patients and healthcare providers regarding communicating about sexuality and intimacy after a cancer diagnosis?

    Go to the Special Queries page in PubMed (http://www.nlm.nih.gov/ bsd/special_queries.html) and click on Health Services Research (HSR) Queries. Enter the terms "cancer sexuality intimacy" in the search window and hit the radio buttons for Qualitative and Narrow, specific search. Click GO. Conducting this search on May 6, 2008, 7 citations are retrieved. Citation #1, PMID 17391082 addresses your question.

SEARCHING EXERCISES FOR CHAPTER 10

Secondary Publications: Systematic Review Articles

1. Does obesity in adults cause depression? This is complex to search because searching cannot easily differentiate between depression causing obesity or obesity causing depression—try to limit your retrievals to those studies in which the obesity came first and caused the depression.

    This again is difficult to search and almost nothing shows up. Good places to try this are in DARE and the TRIP databases. TRIP provides the citation below, which is probably the strongest review article on the topic. From this review, weak evidence seems to indicate that obesity is linked to increased depression later in life.

    DARE: http://www.crd.york.ac.uk/crdweb/

    TRIP: http://www.tripdatabase.com/index.html

    Atlantis E, Baker M. Obesity effects on depression: systematic review of epidemiological studies. Int J Obes (Lond). 2008 Jun;32(6):881-91.

2. Sugar-sweetened beverages, and lots of them, have had a place in many of the lives of our adolescents. Is the consumption of sugar-sweetened beverages associated with obesity in adolescents or children?

    In PubMed using the following search terms, "sugar sweetened beverages obesity meta-analysis" one meta-analysis is obtained on January 15, 2009:

    Forshee RA, Anderson PA, Storey ML. Sugar-sweetened beverages and body mass index in children and adolescents: a meta-analysis. Am J Clin Nutr. 2008 Jun;87(6):1662-71. Comment in: Am J Clin Nutr. 2008 Nov;88(5):1450-1; author reply 1451-2.

    Forshee et al conclude that analysis of both qualitative and quantitative data show that the association between sugar sweetened beverage consumption and body mass index was almost non-existent.

SEARCHING EXERCISES FOR CHAPTER 11

Secondary Publications: Clinical Practice Guidelines

1. Many national and international guidelines exist that mention literacy as being important to health and wellness. Do any guidelines exist that concentrate only on literacy? If so, what countries do they represent? Try the MEDLINE and any other source you can think of.

The first line of approach to finding guidelines is to use the US National Guidelines Clearinghouse (http://www.guideline.gov/).

As of January 15, 2009 20 guidelines in the NGC mention literacy. Of note are several from the Care for the Homeless Clinicians' Network, National Health Care for the Homeless Council. None deal solely with literacy.

The Canadian Medical Association database of clinical practice guidelines includes one guideline specifically on literacy:

http://www.cps.ca/English/statements/PP/pp06-01.htm

Read, speak, sing: Promoting literacy in the physician's office Psychosocial Paediatrics Committee, Canadian Paediatric Society (CPS)

2. Go the U.S. National Guidelines Clearinghouse and find 2 guidelines that deal with palliative care for patients with heart failure. Work through the screens and "compare" these 2. See if you can discern differences in their development and if these differences have any affect on the recommendations.

SEARCHING EXERCISES FOR CHAPTER 12

Secondary Publications: Economic Analyses

1. Is aspirin cost effective in the primary prevention of cardiovascular disease in women?

    Go to the Special Queries page in PubMed (http://www.nlm.nih.gov/bsd/special_queries.html) and click on Health Services Research (HSR) Queries. Enter the terms "aspirin cardiovascular disease women" in the search window and hit the radio buttons for Economics and Narrow, specific search. Click GO. Conducting this search on May 16, 2008, 78 citations are retrieved. Citation #7, PMID 17296886 addresses your question.

2. Is an adjuvant treatment course of spa treatment compared with usual care only cost effective in patients with fibromyalgia syndrome?

    Go to the Special Queries page in PubMed (http://www.nlm.nih.gov/bsd/special_queries.html) and click on Health Services Research (HSR) Queries. Enter the terms "spa treatment fibromyalgia" in the search window and hit the radio buttons for Qualitative and Broad, sensitive search. Click GO. Conducting this search on May 16, 2008, 1 citation is retrieved, PMID 17636181, which addresses your question.

SEARCHING EXERCISES FOR CHAPTER 13

Secondary Publications: Health Technology Assessment

1. Determine how many counties have completed HTAs on the use of portable home dialysis units. Do they have conflicting recommendations?

   The Database of Reviews of Effects at the University of York and its component database of HTAs include several on home dialysis ("home dialysis" in the search window). Canada, the United Kingdom, and Denmark have published substantial HTA reports on the topic.

   http://www.crd.york.ac.uk/CRDWeb/search.aspx?SessionID=858802&SearchID=858802&SearchFor=home+dialysis&RPP=10&DB=HTA&DefaultOr=No&D=7&E=40&H=6

Secondary Publications: Health Technology Assessment

Index

Note: Page numbers with "*t*" denote tables.